Cambridge Elements ☰

Elements of Improving Quality and Safety in Healthcare
edited by
Mary Dixon-Woods,* Katrina Brown,* Sonja Marjanovic,†
Tom Ling,† Ellen Perry,* and Graham Martin*
*THIS Institute (The Healthcare Improvement Studies Institute)
†RAND Europe

REDUCING OVERUSE

Caroline Cupit, Carolyn Tarrant, and Natalie Armstrong

Department of Health Sciences, University of Leicester

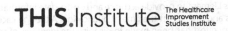

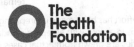

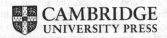

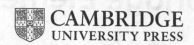

CAMBRIDGE
UNIVERSITY PRESS

Shaftesbury Road, Cambridge CB2 8EA, United Kingdom

One Liberty Plaza, 20th Floor, New York, NY 10006, USA

477 Williamstown Road, Port Melbourne, VIC 3207, Australia

314–321, 3rd Floor, Plot 3, Splendor Forum, Jasola District Centre,
New Delhi – 110025, India

103 Penang Road, #05–06/07, Visioncrest Commercial, Singapore 238467

Cambridge University Press is part of Cambridge University Press & Assessment,
a department of the University of Cambridge.

We share the University's mission to contribute to society through the pursuit of
education, learning and research at the highest international levels of excellence.

www.cambridge.org
Information on this title: www.cambridge.org/9781009310680

DOI: 10.1017/9781009310642

First published 2023

A catalogue record for this publication is available from the British Library.

ISBN 978-1-009-31068-0 Paperback
ISSN 2754-2912 (online)
ISSN 2754-2904 (print)

Reducing Overuse

Elements of Improving Quality and Safety in Healthcare

DOI: 10.1017/9781009310642
First published online: January 2023

Caroline Cupit, Carolyn Tarrant, and Natalie Armstrong
Department of Health Sciences, University of Leicester

Author for correspondence: Natalie Armstrong,
natalie.armstrong@leicester.ac.uk

Abstract: Overuse has become a major issue of healthcare quality, safety, and sustainability around the world. In this Element, the authors discuss concepts, terminology, and the history of concerns. They show how interventions to address overuse target multiple drivers. They highlight not only successes and promising approaches but also challenges in generating and using evidence about overuse. They emphasise that different stakeholder perceptions of value must be recognised. System-level efforts to restrict access to services have created tensions between stakeholder groups and stimulated politicised debates about rationing. They argue for clear articulation of priorities, problem definition, mechanisms for interventions, and areas of uncertainty. Policy-makers should prioritise transparency, be alert to inequalities as they seek to reduce overuse, and consider how to balance controlling use with enabling clinicians to respond to individual circumstances. The complexity of the drivers and possible solutions to overuse require the use of multiple research methods, including social science studies. This title is also available as Open Access on Cambridge Core.

Keywords: overuse, over-diagnosis, low-value care, too much medicine, over-treatment

ISBNs: 9781009310680 (PB), 9781009310642 (OC)
ISSNs: 2754-2912 (online), 2754-2904 (print)

Contents

1 Introduction

Overuse involves the oversupply of interventions beyond the needs of the population. It has become increasingly recognised as a problem of health-care quality,[1–4] where quality refers to 'the degree of match between health products and services, on the one hand, and the needs they are intended to meet, on the other'.[5] In this Element, we explore how concepts related to overuse have been variously employed across research, policy-making, and clinical practice. We highlight that much work to date has focused on *identifying* overuse rather than examining potential solutions to combat it – but show that even identifying overuse is not straightforward. We describe how overuse is becoming seen as a new 'quality frontier'[5] and explain the challenges in designing and evaluating approaches to improvement. We discuss critiques highlighting the tension between standardised restrictive policies and individualised clinical care.

2 What Is Overuse?

Overuse has been defined as 'the provision of medical services that are more likely to cause harm than good'[6] and accordingly as a form of inappropriate care.[7] Since the adoption of the term by the Institute of Medicine National Roundtable on Health Care Quality in 1998,[8] overuse has increasingly encompassed a range of concepts, including overdiagnosis,[9] overtreatment,[10] and too much medicine.[11,12] It is also often linked with the concept of low-value care. However, overuse and low-value care have different origins and are traceable to different research literatures: research on overuse originated in the clinical community and has been focused on clinically orientated concerns;[8,13] research on low-value care originated with economists and has been focused on improving system-level value.[7,14] Concepts of low-value care in the literature are therefore often broader than those of overuse and based on priority-setting and the comparative cost-effectiveness of interventions – which may result in the classification of interventions that have significant clinical benefit as low-value due to their relative cost.[15,16]

In this Element we focus on overuse of healthcare interventions, broadly defined as diagnoses and treatment interventions that have negligible or no benefit to individuals and that have the potential to cause either direct harm (e.g. side effects) or other unwelcome consequences (e.g. financial or other burden of treatment) for patients, *as well as* wasting resources at a system or societal level.[17,18] We show that there are many challenges in identifying, defining, and measuring overuse, and highlight that all definitions of overuse incorporate both clinical *and* economic concerns to some extent.

3 Understanding Overuse

Overuse can be broadly understood as the provision of interventions that have negligible or no benefit (and may cause harm) to particular groups of patients. However, despite its apparent conceptual simplicity, the term has been used in different ways in different contexts, sometimes bringing together divergent and potentially competing ideas. Research, policy, and practice in this area have all suffered from a lack of consensus on conceptualisation, definition, and measurement, leading to challenges for stakeholders trying to strategically understand and address overuse.

Several conceptual frameworks for understanding overuse have been developed. For example, Lipitz-Snyderman and Bach[19] propose attention to: trade-offs between benefits and harms, and between benefits and costs; and patient preferences (i.e. where these may be inconsistent with evidence or clinical recommendations). Chan et al.[20] suggest that there should be differentiation between 'specific clinical situations or indications for which a service is considered inappropriate or of questionable clinical value' and 'services that may be appropriate for a specific population, such as a high-risk population, but [are] inappropriate or of negligible clinical benefit when applied to other, particularly lower-risk populations'.

Verkerk et al.[21] develop such ideas into a broad typology of low-value care, which reflects medical, system, and patient perspectives.

(1) **Ineffective care:** from a medical perspective, care that is ineffective (in terms of clinical benefit and/or cost) for a certain condition or subgroup of patients, according to scientific standards. Examples include antibiotics for a viral infection or routine echocardiography for asymptomatic patients.
(2) **Inefficient care:** from a societal (or system-level) perspective, care that involves 'inefficient provision or inappropriate high intensity or duration'. Examples include duplication of diagnostic tests and removing stitches in hospital instead of general practice. This form of care may be effective clinically but is also considered as overuse.
(3) **Unwanted care:** from a patient perspective, care that 'does not solve the individual patient's problem or does not fit the individual patient's preferences'. Examples include chemotherapy for a patient who prefers palliative care, or surgery for a patient who prefers conservative treatment.

3.1 Scientific Evidence of Clinical Ineffectiveness

Ineffective care can be considered as one key dimension of overuse. However, establishing unequivocal evidence of clinical ineffectiveness for particular

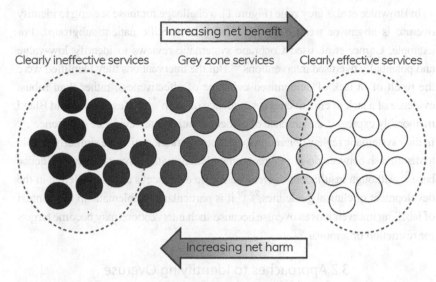

Figure 1 Grey zone services

Reprinted from The Lancet, Brownlee et al.,[6] copyright 2017, with permission from Elsevier. The figure has been published under a non-open-access (standard) licence and permissions for further reuse must be obtained from Elsevier, the holder of the exclusive rights.

interventions and specific patient groups is rarely easy.[21] As Elshaug et al. point out in their report of 150 potentially low-value practices, 'services that are ineffective and/or unsafe across the entire patient population to which they are applied are probably quite rare'.[22] Instead, overuse occurs along a continuum, running from 'universal benefit' to 'entirely ineffective' (see Figure 1):

> *At one end of the continuum lie tests and treatments that are universally beneficial when used on the appropriate patient, such as blood cultures in a young, otherwise healthy patient with sepsis, and insulin for patients with Type 1 diabetes. At the other end of the continuum are services that are entirely ineffective, futile, or pose such a high risk of harm to all patients that they should never be delivered, such as the drug combination fenfluramine-phentermine for obesity. However, the majority of tests and treatments fall into a more ambiguous grey zone.[6]*

To date, a large proportion of the work to identify and address overuse has focused on the 'easy hits'[23] – that is, those interventions with a relatively uncontentious scientific evidence base to demonstrate that they are 'entirely ineffective' for all, or distinct groups of, patients. But as efforts to identify overuse have become more extensive (moving beyond unambiguous cases and into the grey zone), disagreement among experts and other stakeholders has increased, with definitions, underlying principles, and interests all being contested.[2,12,24]

In Brownlee et al.'s grey zone (Figure 1), a challenge for those seeking to identify overuse is absent or weak evidence relating to specific patient subgroups. For example, Garner et al. used Cochrane systematic reviews to identify low-value and potentially overused interventions.[25] But the interventions they identified were the result of 'a lack of randomised evidence of effectiveness, rather than robust evidence of a lack of effectiveness or evidence of harm'[25] – or as Altman and Bland memorably express it, an 'absence of evidence' rather than 'evidence of absence'.[26] In their systematic review of nursing guidelines, Verkerk et al. were similarly unable to distinguish between do-not-do recommendations with a strong or weak evidence base.[27] Although insufficient or weak scientific evidence is also a challenge in the development of clinical guidelines,[28,29] it is particularly problematic in the context of labelling interventions as overuse because such interventions may become targets for restriction or removal.

3.2 Approaches to Identifying Overuse

In addition to the challenges in establishing which interventions might be ineffective and thus vulnerable to overuse, methods for identifying when overuse is occurring in health systems are also diverse and lacking in consensus. One of the most widely used is the RAND Appropriateness Method, which was developed in the USA in the 1980s[8,13] in response to two main issues. First, a recognition of the limited specificity of clinical guidelines, which may recommend that an intervention is considered for a particular group of patients, but not address the conditions under which people within this group may derive limited benefit or experience harm.[30] Second, a new awareness of large geographical variations in the use of some interventions.[31] The RAND approach uses similar techniques to the guideline development process, integrating scientific evidence with the opinions of experts,[1,32] but it also incorporates detailed assessments about the 'appropriateness of performing the procedure for a comprehensive set of specific clinical circumstances or clinical scenarios'.[31]

Other approaches involve systematically reviewing the research evidence for individual conditions. In the UK, for instance, the National Institute for Health and Care Excellence (NICE) has developed do-not-do recommendations based on reviews of clinical guidelines.[33] Its do-not-do database stipulates, for example, that pharmacological intervention should not be employed to aid sleep 'unless sleep problems persist despite following a sleep plan'.[34] Researchers have also undertaken marginal analyses,[35] revisited previous systematic reviews (that were originally focused on intervention rather than potential for overuse),[25] and reassessed health technology assessments.[36–38]

Practice variation studies,[39,40] which seek to identify clinical practices that vary by country, region, or individual clinician, also have a role in assessing overuse. Such studies can provide insight into potential areas of overuse (or underuse) by identifying large geographical differences between and within countries to prioritise opportunities for disinvestment.[41,42] Their premise is that variation is not only due to different population characteristics, but also reflects 'professional uncertainty' – that is, variation in clinicians' beliefs about the outcomes of alternative treatments.[43] Findings can operate as 'tin-openers' – providing data from which to start the process of assessing and making decisions about overuse and underuse.[44] For example, an Australian report based on Organisation for Economic Co-operation and Development data aimed to 'stimulate a national discussion' about whether variation in several orthopaedic, obstetric, and cardiac procedures was warranted.[45] National and international surveillance programmes on antibiotic use are another important example of extensive infrastructure being put in place to enable variation modelling.[46,47] However, interventions with high levels of practice variation are often those for which the current evidence 'does not point clearly to a right answer'[6] on which practice is most effective, thereby creating space for different professional opinions and use of discretionary care.

Practical difficulties in trying to characterise overuse arise because of lack of data in relation to subgroups of patients,[20] problems separating data from routine data sources,[1] and a lack of relevant clinical data about symptoms and physical exam findings in electronic health records and administrative databases.[48] The incompleteness of data records has also created significant challenges with interpreting evidence of overuse from one healthcare setting to another.[25] As electronic records make data more accessible, and suites of local indicators are developed based on evidence of overuse from professional societies and campaigns,[49–52] some of these challenges are being addressed. Researchers are increasingly using new methods to identify overuse within healthcare systems – for example by using algorithms to interrogate administrative databases.[50] In line with the underpinning scientific evidence and focus of professional campaigns such as Choosing Wisely, such work has been orientated towards tests and procedures rather than, for instance, prescribing.[53]

3.3 Determining Overuse in the Context of Differing Perceptions of Value

The approaches for identifying overuse highlighted in Section 3.2 are typically based on research evidence of clinical and cost-effectiveness,[54,55] which is consistent with the argument that 'only evidence from clinical research has secure standing as knowledge'.[56] But the methods for producing standardised evidence for application in clinical practice are, of course, open to challenge.[28,57–60] Increasingly, tensions are being recognised between standardised systems for assessing overuse and clinical judgements when applied in context. For policy-makers, determining the *value* of interventions requires more than scientific measures of effectiveness in the treatment of individual conditions: it also involves complex and context-dependent decisions about options, and allocative concepts of value – 'health outcomes achieved per dollar spent'.[14]

At this system and policy level, there is frequent tension between financial and quality imperatives.[61] Concepts of low value in this context include considerations of the *comparative value* of interventions given restricted budgets and allocative options, which may go beyond strictly clinical/scientific concepts. Healthcare commissioners may come under pressure, for reasons of cost, to restrict interventions and services that have been approved as clinically evidence-based.[62] By the same token, decisions about overuse may be influenced by the range of alternatives that are available and their associated costs and burdens. For example, surgery for minimally symptomatic inguinal hernia could be considered as overuse,[63] since this condition can be managed effectively with so-called watchful waiting. But this alternative strategy also requires clinical activity and resources, so the decision may not be straightforward. More generally, comparing surgical interventions with more conservative options (e.g. physiotherapy) is often more complex than it might initially appear, complicating assessments of overuse.

Determining value may also involve considering the (potentially conflicting) interests of different stakeholders. Antibiotic overuse is a particularly complex area: as well as debates about what constitutes appropriate use in clinical practice,[64] there is difficulty in balancing the value of antibiotics to individual patients in the short term against the longer-term risk to society of growing antimicrobial resistance. Controversies about managing antibiotic overuse point to the need for both responsible use in terms of optimising clinical outcomes, and broader stewardship programmes that protect the efficacy of antibiotics for wider society and patients of the future.[65]

Further complexity arises when the views of patients and the public are factored into thinking about what counts as overuse. An increasingly influential view is that identifying an intervention as low value should be based on the features of the individual encounter, rather than done in a general way outside of a specific situation.[66] This and similar arguments emphasise that individual patient needs and preferences should be core to decision-making about the value of interventions in practice.[59,67,68] In this individualised context, the most important outcomes for some patients may diverge from those that are prioritised within the scientific frame of knowledge[69] (see Box 1). While patients may in many cases opt for more conservative options when informed about the likelihood of benefits and potential harms,[74] this approach can be problematic if patients seek interventions that are not deemed appropriate within the healthcare system. This can be seen in public calls for population-based screening programmes for conditions for which existing research evidence does not support screening, for example.

Ultimately, identifying what is deemed appropriate use cannot be seen as an entirely scientific or neutral enterprise. Instead, it is a social process with multiple political, economic, and relational dimensions[75,76] (see Box 2). Despite Porter's argument that a scientific and economically calculated 'value

---

BOX 1 BALANCING THE POSSIBLE BENEFITS AND HARMS OF BREAST CANCER SCREENING

Screening for breast cancer with mammography is often discussed in the overdiagnosis and overtreatment literature. This is because of its tendency to identify anomalies that would not have gone on to cause a problem for the individual concerned, but are then subject to intervention.

A 2011 Cochrane review of breast screening suggested that for 2,000 women screened over a period of 10 years, one would have her life prolonged but an additional 10 would be treated unnecessarily.[70] In 2012, the Independent UK Panel on Breast Cancer Screening came to the view that while screening did reduce breast cancer mortality, there was an associated cost of overdiagnosis for other screening participants.[71] The review placed the figure at about three overdiagnosed cases identified and treated for every one breast cancer death prevented.

The balance between possible benefits and harms has led to calls for better information for those invited to take part in breast screening – in particular, for information clearly stating the potential for overdiagnosis and subsequent overtreatment. In Australia, a randomised controlled trial of a decision aid including information on overdiagnosis to support informed choice about breast cancer screening[72] suggested that the additional information increased the number of women making an informed choice about whether or not to have screening. It also indicated that being better informed *might* mean women were less likely to be screened. However, other work (by several of the same authors) on women's harm/benefit trade-offs has suggested that people have high tolerance for overdiagnosis, with around half of women reporting that they would always be screened, even at a 6:1 overdiagnosis-to-death-avoided ratio.[73]

Box 2 Controversies in defining appropriate use — an example
from cardiovascular disease prevention

Controversies around defining and identifying overuse are particularly
evident in debates around the use of preventative medications in healthy
people. In recent years, medications targeting cardiovascular risk conditions (e.g. hypertension, type 2 diabetes mellitus) or calculations of overall
risk have become a key feature of cardiovascular disease prevention.[77–79]
The widespread prescription of these interventions for primary prevention
(i.e. to people without history of cardiovascular disease) is intended to
save both lives and money.[80] For example, the National Health Service
(NHS) Health Check programme, which has operated in England since
2009, aims to address underuse of preventative medications by identifying
people to whom they should be prescribed, and quality measures in
general practice incentivise such prescribing.[81]

However, the widespread use of these preventative medications and
apparently rigid adherence to guidelines in this area have been
challenged.[82] Some clinical leaders claim that preventative medications
may do more harm than good, with side effects outweighing potential
predicted future benefits in many cases and broader harms (e.g. psychological, treatment burden) emerging from diagnostic labelling.[83,84] The
widely publicised controversy over statin medications (coined the 'statin
wars') illustrates such contentions,[85] with critics highlighting their widespread prescription as a case of overuse rather than underuse.[86,87] Others
have disputed the value of the NHS Health Check programme, arguing
that it diverts resources to population groups in least need.[88]

At the heart of the debate are competing framings of the benefits and
harms of medications and ideas about how standardised knowledge from
research and guidelines should be translated into practice.

for patients' should take precedence over the 'myriad, often conflicting goals' of
stakeholders,[14] the practices involved in identifying overuse (and underuse) are
inevitably complex and social. Overuse has been related to payment systems
(e.g. fee for service), but also to interrelated patient, clinician, and healthcare
system factors. Patterns of overuse can be surprising when, for example, system
change shapes new behaviours.[89]

3.4 Recognising Overuse as a Quality Problem

Notwithstanding the debates about defining and measuring it, overuse is
increasingly seen as a problem for health systems, populations, and patients.

Researchers have estimated that 'around 20% of mainstream clinical practice brings no benefit to the patient'.[90] Although such estimates are largely based on the US healthcare system, researchers working in other countries have reported similar findings. An international review of overuse estimates that 'approximately a third of all patients (between 20% and 33%, depending on the study), receive treatments or services that the evidence suggests are unnecessary, ineffective or potentially harmful'.[91] Individual studies suggest rates of overuse may be very much higher for some interventions, in some contexts – with one study in China finding that 57% of patients had been prescribed inappropriate antibiotics.[5]

Overuse has sometimes been identified as a particular problem in high-income countries,[6,32] but patterns of overuse – and underuse – are not always simple. In 2017, *The Lancet* published a series of articles on 'right care', based on studies of overuse around the world.[4–6,92–95] It highlighted that overuse and underuse (the latter defined as 'the failure to use effective and affordable medical interventions'[94]) were both widespread and should be understood and addressed in parallel.[92] Overuse and underuse may coexist within the same health economies, across the spectrum of different intervention types and/or for a single intervention across different patient groups. Overuse and underuse may be present in both high-income and low-income countries. Overuse has been (and continues to be) a persistent challenge even in low-income countries and in communities with limited access to healthcare services, where overuse may be a response to poor living conditions or limitations of available healthcare services.[5,96,97]

Concerns about overuse have become increasingly prominent in the healthcare community, particularly as increasing numbers of studies show that overuse has potentially major consequences for patients – including costs, emotional distress and anxiety, physical harms from side effects, or other adverse events[9,83,98–100] – and for the sustainability of healthcare systems.[3,101] Addressing overuse has recently been positioned as a new 'quality frontier' in international work to improve healthcare quality,[5] being linked with the Institute of Medicine's dimensions of quality.[102,103] Increasingly, it has been positioned as a patient safety ('harm') issue,[100] stretching the concept of safety to include psychological harm as well as physical injury.[104]

3.5 Recognising Systemic Influences on Overuse

To address overuse as a systemic quality issue, it is necessary to have an appreciation of its systemic drivers (Figure 2). For example, efforts to address problems of *underuse* may unintentionally result in *overuse*.[98,105] Clinical guidelines provide

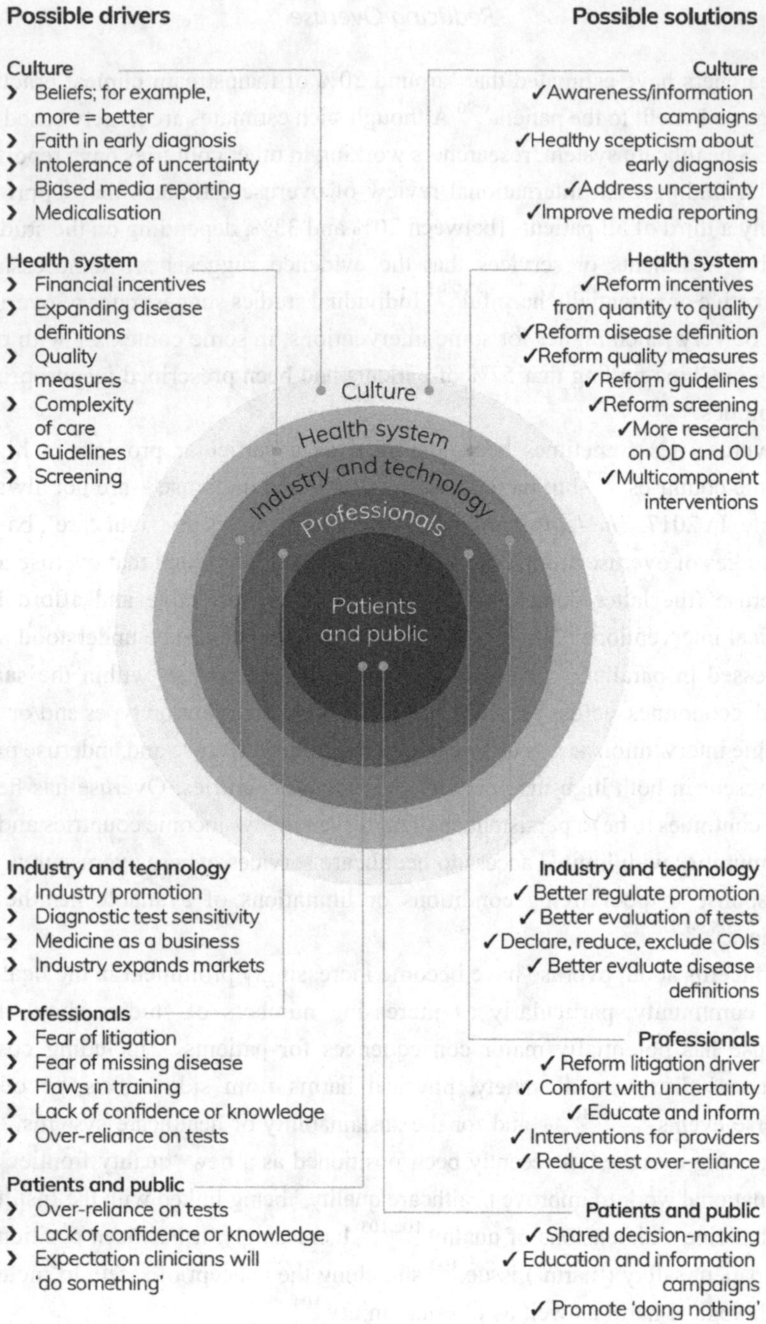

Possible drivers

Culture
> Beliefs; for example, more = better
> Faith in early diagnosis
> Intolerance of uncertainty
> Biased media reporting
> Medicalisation

Health system
> Financial incentives
> Expanding disease definitions
> Quality measures
> Complexity of care
> Guidelines
> Screening

Industry and technology
> Industry promotion
> Diagnostic test sensitivity
> Medicine as a business
> Industry expands markets

Professionals
> Fear of litigation
> Fear of missing disease
> Flaws in training
> Lack of confidence or knowledge
> Over-reliance on tests

Patients and public
> Over-reliance on tests
> Lack of confidence or knowledge
> Expectation clinicians will 'do something'

Possible solutions

Culture
✓ Awareness/information campaigns
✓ Healthy scepticism about early diagnosis
✓ Address uncertainty
✓ Improve media reporting

Health system
✓ Reform incentives from quantity to quality
✓ Reform disease definition
✓ Reform quality measures
✓ Reform guidelines
✓ Reform screening
✓ More research on OD and OU
✓ Multicomponent interventions

Industry and technology
✓ Better regulate promotion
✓ Better evaluation of tests
✓ Declare, reduce, exclude COIs
✓ Better evaluate disease definitions

Professionals
✓ Reform litigation driver
✓ Comfort with uncertainty
✓ Educate and inform
✓ Interventions for providers
✓ Reduce test over-reliance

Patients and public
✓ Shared decision-making
✓ Education and information campaigns
✓ Promote 'doing nothing'

Culture
Health system
Industry and technology
Professionals
Patients and public

Figure 2 Overdiagnosis and related overuse: mapping possible drivers to potential solutions

Adapted from Pathirana et al.,[105] copyright 2017, with permission from BMJ Publishing Group Ltd; permission conveyed through Copyright Clearance Center, Inc. The figure has been published under a non-open-access (standard) licence and permissions for further reuse must be obtained from BMJ Publishing Group Ltd, the holder of the exclusive rights. COI = conflict of interest; OD = overdiagnosis; OU = overuse.

a clear example: historically, they focused on what *should* be done rather than what *should not* be done (and in what circumstances).[98] Associated payment models and other (e.g. reputational) incentives have not always targeted the *appropriate* use of interventions, but they have influenced physicians' recommendations and so may lead to a situation of oversupply.[106] Less obvious systemic features, such as appointment structures that fail to allow enough time for thorough explanations of the benefits and harms of potential interventions, may also contribute to overuse. Other drivers relate to frontline interactions between professionals and patients (e.g. cultural beliefs that more is better,[105,107] defensive medicine, lack of recognition of the potential harms and limits of medical interventions), and market factors (e.g. industry-driven new technologies).[105,107] The widespread overuse of knee arthroscopy in conditions such as knee arthritis and meniscal tears provides an example of how various drivers converge to produce overuse. Its overuse has been attributed to patient expectations, financial incentives, and patients or clinicians erroneously attributing clinical improvements following surgery to the arthroscopy intervention, rather than to other factors.[107]

Even apparently individualised behaviours are shaped systemically[105] and are not simply the result of individual choices. For example, professionals' fear of litigation is directly linked to the institutional systems through which they are monitored and held accountable. Clinicians may err on the side of caution, proceeding with interventions of unclear utility in an effort to fit in with local practice and customs and to help them defend themselves should questions be asked about their practice.[108] And a survey of US physicians found that respondents reported that colleagues were 'more likely to perform unnecessary procedures when they profit from them'.[109] Overuse may also become normalised and embedded in policies and guidelines over time due to oversupply[110] – with or without involvement of conflicts of interest that are known to distort healthcare research, strategy, expenditure, and practice.[111] Multiple and intersecting drivers arising from different parts of the healthcare system precipitate ethical questions about who is accountable for overuse and its prevention – for example, individual clinicians, healthcare managers, or politicians?

4 Efforts to Address Overuse

Efforts to address overuse come in many different shapes and sizes. It is not possible to cover all of these in detail but, in this section, we present an overview of the international literature using illustrative examples to demonstrate a selection of types of activities and some of the challenges involved. Many of our examples are drawn from the UK, with its distinctive health system characteristics. Interventions elsewhere have similarly been shaped by their own healthcare contexts, particularly the payment mechanisms involved and wider drivers of overuse that dominate the healthcare landscape.

4.1 Campaigns and Awareness-Raising Activities

Advocacy activity and campaigns increasingly target the problem of overuse, united by the goal of achieving widespread reduction in the use of ineffective or inappropriate interventions, based on established scientific evidence. This activity has drawn attention to a range of interventions, including tests, treatments, and processes of care that are argued to have questionable or no benefit and which should therefore be avoided or withdrawn.[6,20,22,112] Overuse campaigns include a series of special issues on 'too much medicine' in the *British Medical Journal*,[113] and the international Preventing Overdiagnosis movement.[9] National campaigns in Scotland (Realistic Medicine[114]) and Wales (Prudent Healthcare[16]) have accompanied those based in England. Elsewhere, initiatives have included the *Journal of the American Medical Association*'s 'less is more' series[19] and *The Lancet's* 'right care' series.[4–6,92–95] Reports from influential healthcare organisations have also brought the topic to greater prominence.[3]

The American Board of Internal Medicine (ABIM) Foundation's Choosing Wisely campaign,[115] which was established in 2012 and arose from work to improve performance of the US healthcare system, is a particularly important campaign internationally in highlighting the potential harms of overuse for patients. Choosing Wisely campaigns in the USA and elsewhere have centred on specific overused tests and interventions (see Box 3 for the UK implementation of the campaign,[75,120] which is led by the Academy of Medical Royal Colleges[116]). In most cases, targeting of these interventions is based on high-quality evidence[121] and on prevalence data indicating significant opportunity to improve care and achieve better value for money.[122]

The Choosing Wisely campaign has taken a bottom-up approach,[91] targeting clinicians, patients, and the public with the aim of 'supporting conversations between physicians and patients about what care is truly necessary'.[123] Patients have been positioned as consumers who can push back against the institutional forces that lead to overuse. In the USA, ABIM's partnership with Consumer Reports (a non-profit consumer organisation) has led to considerable success in reaching into the public domain with educational messages relating to overuse.[48,123] The campaign has simultaneously adapted its message to appeal to clinicians by framing overuse as a problem of waste as well as unnecessary and potentially harmful treatment.[123]

> ### Box 3 Choosing Wisely and other UK campaigns
>
> The UK's Choosing Wisely campaign[116] has published a list of 40 over-used interventions that patients and clinicians should question.[117] It has also developed resources for patients and clinicians to support shared decision-making, such as 'Four questions to ask my clinician or nurse to make better decisions together', which uses the acronym BRAN:
>
> - What are the Benefits?
> - What are the Risks?
> - What are the Alternatives?
> - What if I do Nothing?
>
> Other national initiatives that have sought to address overuse include Realistic Medicine (Scotland) and Prudent Healthcare (Wales). These national healthcare strategies[114,118] provide overarching principles[119] around which a wide range of improvement activities (more or less geared to overuse) have been aligned. The principles emphasise that many patients prefer less intervention than they receive and stress the need for improved shared decision-making (see Box 5). As with the campaigns Choosing Wisely and Preventing Overdiagnosis, these UK-based national strategy ambitions have not always been subject to robust evaluation either prior to or alongside their implementation.

Studies of US commercial insurance claims data thus far have concluded that Choosing Wisely has had only a marginal impact on its targeted interventions.[124,125] But Bhatia et al. suggest a broader 'integrative framework' approach to evaluating outcomes is needed, including clinical measures from electronic records alongside patient and physician experience surveys and patient-reported outcome measures.[126] However, as Chalmers et al.[51] have subsequently reported, the vast majority of recommendations from the Choosing Wisely lists are not measurable using routinely collected datasets, leading to considerable complexities in meaningfully measuring outcomes.

The international Preventing Overdiagnosis campaign has also provided a focus for clinicians and researchers committed to reducing the use of ineffect-ive or harmful interventions. Like Choosing Wisely, its goals have been primar-ily around articulating and drawing attention to the problem and gaining support among clinicians. Since 2013, the campaign's annual conference has high-lighted the harms associated with early detection and the widening of disease definitions, thereby providing a counter-narrative to the dominant surveillance-focused narratives embedded in health policy.[9] Such high-profile forums have been supported by ground-level movements such as the Royal College of General Practitioners' overdiagnosis group,[127] which has provided day-to-day opportunities for general practitioners (GPs) and others to discuss the science and the practicalities around issues of overdiagnosis.

4.2 Tackling Overuse through Different Approaches to Care

Although the problem of overuse has been recognised in research and policy domains for several decades, until recently many efforts to tackle it have been relatively 'passive'.[128–130] These have included the publication of guidelines or educational materials,[130] health technology reassessment outputs such as NICE's do-not-do lists,[131,132] evolution in prescribing patterns,[128] and other evidence of a practice's ineffectiveness or harm.[129] Some of these approaches have had a significant impact on practice.[133] But in this section we focus mainly on what some have described as 'active strategies to change practices'.[130] These more active strategies go beyond awareness-raising, the dissemination of tools and guidelines, and educational or decision support. They involve the types of intervention that are commonly understood as quality improvement – usually incorporating defined mechanisms, theories of change, and outcome measures.

Verkerk et al. have argued that understanding the different types of low-value care is fundamental to tackling overuse effectively.[21] They suggest (Figure 3) three broad approaches: ineffective care requires a 'limit' approach, inefficient care requires a 'lean' approach, and unwanted care requires a 'listen' approach. (For further details on Lean approaches to improving quality and safety in healthcare, see the Element on Lean and associated techniques for process improvement.[134])

Internationally, the majority of interventions targeting overuse have fallen into Verkerk's 'limit' category, most commonly targeting medication use (56%), followed by radiology (12%), procedures (10%), and labs/pathology (10%).[133] Colla et al. found that most interventions were implemented in hospitals (56%), followed by ambulatory care settings (20%) and health systems (16%).[133] They identified a variety of both demand-side and supply-side interventions. On the demand side, interventions included patient cost-sharing (i.e. where the cost of healthcare services is divided between the patient and the insurance plan), patient education, and public reporting of provider performance. On the supply side were interventions such as pay-for-performance, insurer restrictions, risk-sharing agreements (which spread the financial and clinical risks from introducing a new drug between the pharmaceutical company and the health authorities), clinical decision support (see

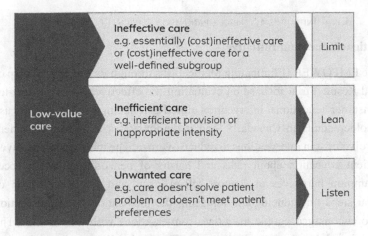

Figure 3 Typology of low-value care
Adapted from Verkerk et al.,[21] in accordance with the terms of the Creative Commons Attribution Licence (https://creativecommons.org/licenses/by/4.0).

Box 4), clinician education, provider feedback, and interventions with multiple elements. Clinician decision-support interventions were most commonly applied in order to limit overuse and were also reported to be most effective.

Although decision-support interventions have been shown to be successful in many contexts, they may be complicated by factors such as difficulty in incorporating standardised protocols into individualised care, and difficulty anticipating the harms from potential interventions due to these occurring further downstream from the unnecessary intervention.[104] Boxes 4–6 highlight some examples of successful interventions to address overuse, as well as the complexities of implementing such interventions that relate to applying evidence in real-world contexts.

Some researchers have argued that interventions should focus more on 'direct intervention by reimbursement policy makers',[128] encouraging policy-makers involved in contract management to use payment systems (which may or may not have been driving overuse) as levers on clinical practice. However, changing payment systems alone is unlikely to address overuse without precipitating detrimental consequences. Increasingly, researchers have highlighted that multiple, interrelated factors *drive* overuse, and that interventions to *address* overuse should therefore reflect these multiple dimensions – which are specific to the particular healthcare context.

Colla et al.'s systematic review identifies that the approaches with the most potential to address low-value care are those that involve multicomponent interventions targeting both patients and clinicians.[133] The review also highlights

Box 4 INITIATIVES TO TRIGGER PATIENT OR CLINICIAN RECONSIDERATION

Patient Education Initiative

The EMPOWER (Eliminating Medications through Patient OWnership of End Results) trial focused on evaluating the effectiveness of a direct-to-consumer educational intervention aimed at reducing benzodiazepine use in older adults in Canada,[135] and it demonstrates the value of patient involvement in interventions to reduce overuse. The intervention involved patient education about risks and harms of benzodiazepine use, peer champion narratives to support self-efficacy, and the specification of clear steps for reducing and replacing the medication. The intervention also encouraged people to initiate conversations with their doctor. The trial found that the intervention was effective in eliciting discussion and shared decision-making, resulting in significant levels of deprescribing and dose reduction.

Implementing an Approval Process before Knee Arthroscopy

Chen et al.'s Australian study involved a clinical governance process which required clinicians to seek approval from a senior clinician prior to referring a patient aged 50 years or older for knee arthroscopy.[136] Although there is strong evidence against undertaking this procedure, referral rates had remained high. Following the intervention, referral rates dropped (by almost 60% in one region), indicating that simple and low-resource policies can have a significant impact on clinician behaviours in some circumstances.

clinical decision support and performance feedback as effective strategies with a sound evidence base. The authors recommend more extensive use and evaluation of multicomponent interventions. Their review also identifies problems and gaps in the research, including publication bias, a focus on volume reduction rather than value, dominance of acute sector interventions, and few studies that include more clinically meaningful measures, such as clinical appropriateness, patient-reported outcomes, or elicited patient preferences.[133,148]

Overall, there is a paucity of good quality literature on interventions to address overuse in low-income and middle-income countries, with obvious implications for addressing urgent problems such as the inappropriate use of antibiotics.[149] In all clinical and geographical contexts, it is important to recognise that, as shown in Figure 2, complex social factors (e.g. antibiotics as a quick fix within a resource-stretched healthcare system[97]) complicate simple concepts of getting evidence into practice. (See the Element on implementation science for a broader discussion.[150])

Box 5 SHARED DECISION-MAKING INTERVENTIONS

Shared decision-making is increasingly being positioned as a means to tackle overuse.[105] A key element is the perceived potential to change the way decisions are framed by signalling that doing nothing or pursuing a strategy of active surveillance (rather than immediate intervention) can be discussed as a deliberate or positive action.[137] By focusing on joint decisions between the patient and clinician, the approach involves both demand-side and supply-side elements.[138]

Shared decision-making has a prominent place in the UK's Choosing Wisely campaign, alongside recommendations for clinicians of things not to do and questions for patients to ask of their clinicians (see Box 3). Shared decision-making is promoted as an effective strategy for tackling overdiagnosis and overtreatment, with Choosing Wisely citing what it sees as its positive influence on inappropriate antibiotic use in acute respiratory infections, for example.

One prominent example is the MAGIC (MAking Good decisions In Collaboration) programme, which ran between 2010 and 2013 as a knowledge translation project designed to test the implementation of shared decision-making in real-world clinical contexts.[139] The programme was based on a large body of evidence showing the benefits of shared decision-making, including its potential impact on overuse[140] – an evidence base that has since been extended.[5,141] MAGIC highlighted various challenges to implementing shared decision-making in practice.[142] These included factors relating to clinicians, patients, and healthcare organisations, summarised as: 'We do it already'; 'We don't have the right tools'; 'Patients don't want shared decision-making'; 'How can we measure it?'; and 'We have too many other demands and priorities'. A particular problem in general practice was that processes for shared decision-making could come into conflict with financial incentives encouraging particular activities. The project also suffered from difficulties in developing meaningful outcome measures.

5 Critiques of Approaches to Addressing Overuse

The analysis presented so far in this Element has emphasised the pressing importance of work to address overuse, both to avoid patient harm and to ensure limited healthcare resources are used wisely, particularly as it is likely that many reports have underestimated the scale of the problem and the diverse harms.

Box 6 Pharmacist roles for deprescribing in care homes

Some efforts to tackle medicines overuse as a system-wide problem have involved investment in new roles to review and optimise medicines use, as well as changes to the organisation and delivery of services. In the UK, these approaches have been used to address problematic polypharmacy, defined as use of multiple medications, where 'the multiple medications are pre-scribed inappropriately, or where the intended benefit of the medication is not realised'.[143] It is associated with risk of harm from adverse drug reactions and other negative outcomes. For older people in particular, it is associated with increased risk of falls, hospital admission, and mortality.

Problematic polypharmacy results from a silo-based, as opposed to holistic, approach to care of people living with multimorbidity. The national NHS England Medicines Optimisation in Care Homes programme[144] involves the creation of new pharmacist roles to support review and optimisation of medicines for older people in care homes. The focus is on reducing unnecessary medication in the context of multidis-ciplinary team-working across primary care and social care settings. Alves et al.'s 5-year evaluation of a pharmacy-led model of deprescribing – a team of primary care pharmacists supported GP practices in Somerset to undertake medication reviews and deprescribing in care homes – found it led to a wide range of pharmacist interventions to deprescribe medications that were deemed not to be needed, or where polypharmacy presented a safety risk. The programme also generated significant cost savings.[145]

A challenge for system-wide approaches targeting deprescribing in care homes is that of overcoming some of the barriers to medication optimisation for this patient group. For older people with dementia and people approaching the end of life, decisions about optimising medication may be complicated by reduced decision-making capacity and difficulties with comprehension and communication. Involving relatives and carers may result in conflicting views, and establishing goals of care may be complex.[146] This highlights the tensions between organisational, regional, or national goals to reduce problematic polypharmacy and aspirations for shared decision-making at the point of care about what might be best for the individual. An example of an approach that aims to support shared decision-making about deprescribing in care home settings is the medica-tion review project, funded by the Health Foundation and led by Northumbria Healthcare NHS Trust, which aimed to put care home residents and their relatives at the centre of the decision-making process.[147]

Approaches to addressing overuse have taken a variety of forms, often targeting the behaviour of clinicians in order to prevent inappropriate care, or promoting shared decision-making in anticipation that this will reduce patient demand for interventions. We have highlighted the growing body of evidence about the effectiveness of approaches to address overuse, which points to the value of multicomponent interventions.

In Section 5.1, we present some prominent critiques that support advances towards greater system-level intervention. Then in Section 5.2, we discuss an alternative and opposing critique that highlights the potential impact of such authoritative policy programmes on stakeholders, importantly frontline clinicians and patients. We highlight that the enthusiasm for the avoidance of harm associated with overuse and for wise use of resources may not always carry over into support for more restrictive approaches that remove (apparently) valid options. In drawing attention to this opposing critique, our aim is not to undermine the importance of finding effective approaches to addressing overuse (all interventions and policies inevitably bring about their own winners and losers); rather, we hope that by highlighting such tensions, we can bring to the fore important social elements of intervention development that may be overlooked – sometimes to the detriment of their success. These critiques prompt our own final reflections on the topic in Section 6.

5.1 Moving towards System-Level Healthcare Improvement

As we noted in Section 3, researchers have increasingly drawn attention to the need to systematically identify and address overuse across whole healthcare systems.[2,20,50,151] Although some impact can be achieved by withdrawing interventions completely from approved treatment protocols, this is appropriate for a minority of interventions only; many interventions may be appropriate in some, but not other, circumstances. In addition, experts have observed that a greater burden of proof is generally required to remove interventions from established guidelines and protocols than it is to incorporate them in the first place.[152]

Nassery et al. propose that creating an index of overused services (similar to a stock market portfolio) would enable policy-makers to identify and address the structural problems that generate overuse. They suggest that such an approach would facilitate a shift from addressing overuse in a 'piecemeal' fashion (i.e. individual clinical topics identified and addressed in isolation) to addressing it as 'a widespread and pervasive phenomenon'.[2] But, as we have seen, the evidence base is skewed towards particular areas of medicine, with more studies in curative medicine, for example, than in rehabilitative care, health promotion, or nursing practice.[27,153] In order to enable more informed prioritisation at a system level, more diversity of studies is required, as is greater transparency about the quality and scope of the available evidence.[153]

Some have advocated more broadly for multicomponent interventions[133] that are carefully integrated into clinical care pathways and include 'policy changes and/or changes to funding models' as these are 'predicted to have the greatest likelihood of facilitating de-adoption'.[129] However, better understanding of the *drivers* of overuse (involving multiple organisational processes as well as individual behaviours) are needed for this kind of system-level action. And as Harvey and McInnes have noted: '. . . the reasons why healthcare professionals continue with practices for which there is little or no supporting evidence are typically complex and include a combination of individual (eg, beliefs about evidence, past experience), interprofessional (eg, influence of peers), and contextual (eg, economic, industry and marketing influences) factors'.[154]

Hensher et al. similarly have drawn on various economic perspectives (health, behavioural, ecological) to highlight the intersecting individual and system drivers of overuse, the dynamics of which will be different in different healthcare contexts; they note also the complexity of addressing these.[18] However, perhaps as a result of this complexity, system-level dimensions of overuse have consistently been overlooked within approaches to addressing overuse (see Box 7), with the problem often 'misconstrued as . . . arising from both physicians' integrity and autonomy rather than arising from system failures'.[30]

While financial levers are clearly important (e.g. financial incentives for patients and/or rewards or penalties for clinicians, clinics, and hospitals[95]), quality improvement approaches[158] – with their attention to healthcare systems and mechanisms of intervention – are likely also to be important in taking forward work to address overuse. Despite the potential, Chassin lamented in 2013 that overuse has been 'almost entirely left out of the quality improvement discourse',[159] and it would seem that not much has changed since then. Publications such as *The Lancet*'s 'right care' series[4-6,92–95] have highlighted overuse as a quality issue, but there are still relatively few examples of interventional studies that aim to address overuse with fully specified theories of change and outcome measures. Indeed, a 2018 review by Parker et al. identified only a small proportion of studies that outlined theoretical mechanisms of de-adoption;[160] and most of those employed psychological theories or behavioural science approaches (e.g. 'nudge interventions'[161]) targeting frontline behaviours rather than more systemic reasons for overuse.

BOX 7 THE POLITICS OF SYSTEM-LEVEL INTERVENTION IN THE UK

Policy-makers have sometimes been reluctant to address overuse overtly. In the UK, for example, local commissioning organisations have tended to allow overused interventions to '"wither on the vine" through lack of use' (as replacement practices evolve, for example), or be discreetly removed or reconfigured during organisational mergers and takeovers.[62]

More deliberate action to identify and address overuse has generally focused on broader disinvestment for the purpose of cost savings. But due to considerable political sensitivities, local policy-makers have often wanted to keep this work under the public radar to avoid raising concerns about rationing.[44,62,155] Such sensitivities may account for researchers reporting 'little evidence of any tools or frameworks to support disinvestment decision-making' in commissioning organisations,[156] with interventions typically being small-scale and based on comparisons of local data with other commissioning regions.[156,157]

5.2 Tensions between Interventions to Tackle Overuse and Individualised Care

While systematic approaches may have a role in addressing structural factors in overuse, some aspects of them are increasingly being challenged by clinicians and patients. Evidence from across a diverse literature indicates that, in practice, it is difficult to develop consensus among stakeholders about what should be classified as overuse.[120] Systems and processes put in place to reduce the use of existing interventions inevitably have consequences for stakeholders, who may, as discussed earlier, have different understandings of what is valuable. As a result, efforts to standardise definitions of overuse (what is, or is not, appropriate for particular groups of patients), and then to enforce compliance, may not be accepted by professionals or patients[48,162–164] (see Box 8).

Resistance from clinicians and patients arises from ongoing tensions between their autonomy (clinical decision-making) and the imposition of standardised rules to address overuse which restricts that autonomy. Contributing to such tensions is the difficulty in applying traditional instruments for changing practice, which display a '[weak] ability to discriminate between inappropriate and appropriate care'.[18] Indeed, there are significant problems with applying average estimates of effects from the populations of clinical trials to individual patients for whom some benefit may exist.[33] Some treatments and conditions may also be soft targets for restriction, due to a lack of evidence or lobbying muscle from patient groups and social judgements about their value (e.g. cosmetic surgery,

Box 8 THE EVIDENCE-BASED INTERVENTIONS PROGRAMME

In England, the Evidence-Based Interventions (EBI) programme, which was established in 2018, aims to 'reduce the number of inappropriate interventions provided on the NHS'.[165] The programme represents a shift in approach from engagement exercises (e.g. Choosing Wisely) and strategic principles (e.g. Prudent Healthcare) to more targeted ('active') initiatives that are integrated into payment systems.[128] Guidance has been issued to clinical commissioning groups[166] – which are organisations that commission primary care services in England – mandating them to restrict interventions listed as inappropriate, including through the use of financial levers to ensure compliance. An initial list of 17 interventions that 'should not be routinely commissioned' (e.g. dilatation and curettage [D&C] for heavy menstrual bleeding) or 'should only be commissioned or performed when specific criteria are met' (e.g. knee arthroscopy for patients with osteoarthritis) was intended to be expanded over time.[167] There is accompanying guidance on items that should no longer be routinely prescribed in primary care.[168]

Although the programme has emphasised that its main objective is clinical improvement (and any associated savings will be reinvested in patient care[169]), critics have argued that it is geared towards delivering cost savings.[170] Its guidance has been challenged by commentators, clinicians, and patients. Specific criticisms relate to the evidence base for restriction (including blanket restriction of some interventions, which is not in line with NICE clinical guidelines or the best interests of patients), the resources required to explain these restrictions in clinical practice, and the consequences for clinician–patient relationships.[170–172] Debates highlight the tensions between different approaches to determining and measuring value (see work by Chalmers et al.,[51] Pandya,[173] and Tsevat and Moriates[174]).

The EBI programme provides an example of how de-implementation (e.g. restricting existing services) may involve fundamentally different challenges from implementation. Disinvestment initiatives such as this, even when based on an apparently relatively strong evidence base, are likely to be contested when applied to frontline clinical practice. Resistance has been particularly strong where attempts to reduce overuse are integrated into broader cost-savings work; policy-makers face charges of 'rationing' – 'the denial of health care that is beneficial but is deemed to be too costly'.[175] This notion has become highly emotive and political, making policy-makers nervous about how disinvestment work will be perceived. Despite attempts to emphasise the quality improvement angle of decommissioning ineffective or harmful interventions, the distinction between addressing overuse and generating cost savings has been difficult to achieve in local policy-making.[176]

Box 9 Independent Funding Request processes

Independent Funding Request (IFR) processes, which have been put in place as a mechanism for determining exceptionality alongside restrictive policies, have raised concerns about equity – with, for example, some patients apparently swaying decisions by harnessing considerable public and pharmaceutical company support in their appeals for expensive cancer drugs.[177] IFR processes involve judgements about who is deserving of a restricted treatment and invite a huge amount of work from both patients and clinicians in making a case for treatment.[178,179] Due to the inherent problems of implementing IFRs, Heale and Syrett[180] have gone as far as claiming that the IFR process is 'unfair, unacceptable, and probably unlawful'. Other work suggests that targeting the overuse of low-value care in too broad and inflexible a manner may also result in the underuse of high-value care by some groups.[126]

---

orthodontics).[33] Restrictive policies have the potential to lead to significant inequity between people who have what could be considered high-status conditions (i.e. well-recognised with strong research funding) or the social resources to self-advocate, and people who are not in this position (see Box 9).

Ellen et al. have argued that 'a comprehensive approach [to overuse] likely lies in synergistic efforts between stakeholders and governments to identify overuse and subsequently undertake collaborative efforts to address it'.[91] Such efforts should take account of multiple dimensions of quality, including those relating to patients, physicians, and organisations and systems, and might be able to harness the support of those campaigning against overuse. However, as Hodgetts et al.[181] found in their study of participatory decision-making about assisted reproductive technologies, such processes are labour-intensive and (politically) sensitive as they 'involve the negotiation of different orders of evidence (empirical, contextual, and anecdotal), indicating a need for higher level discussion around "what counts and how to count it" when making disinvestment decisions'.

Crucially, patient experiences and patient and public priorities have been largely left out of interventional studies to address overuse systematically:[133,182]

this has meant that harms of overuse (and consequences of restrictive interventions) may be much more extensive than commonly reported, and underlying questions of value may sometimes only emerge during the translation of evidence into policy-making and clinical practice.[182] Although in theory patient perspectives are central to concepts such as value-based healthcare,[174] in practice these concepts are almost entirely economically focused and tend to be derived from the US healthcare context. The lack of focus on patients has led to increasing calls for overuse to be addressed within existing structures for patient safety.[100] Lipitz-Snyderman and Korenstein argue that this has various advantages – in particular, 'framing overuse through the lens of patient safety' provides the issue with an 'institutional home' and helps to highlight overuse 'as an issue that affects clinical outcomes that are most important to patients and clinicians'.[104] However, greater social science analysis is needed to understand overuse, value, and restrictive practices from alternative (particularly under-represented patient) standpoints.[183]

6 Conclusions

In this Element we have highlighted how the term overuse can include a range of related concepts and that these have been variously employed across research, policy-making, and clinical practice. Concerns about overuse are present across a wide variety of healthcare contexts, and we have drawn on diverse examples to demonstrate this. But we have also noted that studies tend to be skewed towards particular areas of medicine, with a larger number of studies in curative medicine rather than in areas such as rehabilitative care, health promotion, or nursing practice.

As we have shown, much work on overuse has been focused on its identification, as this is a logical first step in the process of addressing it. But identifying overuse is not straightforward. We have drawn attention to some of the key challenges involved, particularly around how evidence of overuse is produced and used, and different stakeholder understandings of value. And we have highlighted that producing good evidence around overuse rates is often challenging. Ideas about what constitutes overuse are always shaped by social systems, and views about the possible benefits and potential harms of any particular intervention – and the most appropriate balance between these – may be challenged by those involved. These challenges apply both to efforts to identify particular instances of overuse and efforts to identify and address the problem at healthcare system level.

We have outlined the recent shift to addressing overuse as a new quality frontier, but we have also highlighted how overuse has long been understood, if somewhat neglected, as a form of inappropriate care (alongside underuse and misuse). We have considered increasing calls for overuse to be addressed more systematically, often involving policy-makers and changes to payment systems, but we have also discussed critiques that draw attention to the tension between standardised restrictive policies and individualised clinical care (and the complex social structures involved). Through case studies of efforts to address overuse in various forms, we have demonstrated some of the challenges involved in doing so.

Our discussion has drawn attention to how lack of conceptual clarity around overuse[184] produces practical tensions – in particular, an overarching tension between frontline and management (or financial) understandings of overuse. We observe that tensions – between frontline-clinical and managerial logics of overuse – relates to both identifying and addressing overuse, and we suggest it is likely to be exacerbated as researchers and policy-makers call for more systemic (standardised and incentivised) approaches. Such a challenge is likely to present differently across different healthcare systems.

The issues we have covered, and our reflections on some of the challenges, suggest a number of directions that further work on overuse could usefully take. First is the need for greater transparency about the quality and scope of the evidence available on overuse. In particular, greater diversity and quality of studies across different healthcare contexts would enable more informed prioritisation at a system level. The development of improved methodologies to identify interventions that have little benefit for patients would be helpful in more clearly establishing the scale of the problem.

Second, many of the interventions seeking to address overuse described in the literature are specific to the healthcare context in which they were situated (most are US-based[135]). The drivers and dynamics of overuse are likely to be different across healthcare systems. For example, guidelines, performance measures, and governance processes may incentivise (over)use, as clinicians' work is often orientated to these in the face of uncertainty; these will be context specific.[185] Work is needed to draw out and understand the particular influences at play in different contexts, and how these influences are exerted, in order to inform decisions about whether strategies that seem to have been successful in one context will translate to another. The role of financial and reputational incentives should be a particular focus for research and intervention in fee-for-service systems.

Third, tensions between different concepts of quality and value among stakeholders should be recognised. Research should include (and prioritise) meaningful clinical measures relating to appropriateness and other outcomes that are important to patients.[148] Although there will always be diverse opinions and priorities, and financial resources will always be limited, recognising the political dimensions of overuse might provide a welcome contribution to informed public discussion.

Finally, insights from healthcare improvement research are likely to be valuable in developing successful efforts to address overuse. These include the need to clearly articulate the problem and the factors driving it, as well as the need to recognise that these may vary in different cases – for example, according to features of the particular clinical context, or the professional or patient groups concerned. Also needed is careful, theory-informed design of interventions with clearly articulated and credible proposed mechanisms through which the desired outcomes will be achieved – along with robust evaluation of efforts to tackle the problem, including qualitative process evaluations capable of producing in-depth and nuanced accounts of whether and how interventions have worked in practice. There is a particular need for social science studies that can establish how concepts of overuse are being developed and employed in practice and the (unintended) consequences.[103]

In conclusion, overuse is a significant issue for the quality, safety, and cost of healthcare, particularly in countries where financial and other drivers exert a significant influence on the use of medical services. Addressing the overuse of medicine is a pressing global priority, and understanding the complexities involved is critical to informing new approaches to tackle it.

7 Further Reading

Articles

- Chassin and Galvin[8] – sets out the background to work on addressing overuse.
- Pathirana et al.[105] – an analysis of the drivers of overuse and related solutions.

Journal Series

- *The Lancet*'s right care series: www.thelancet.com/series/right-care.
- *BMJ*'s too much medicine series: www.bmj.com/specialties/too-much-medicine.
- *JAMA*'s less is more series: https://jamanetwork.com/collections/44045/less-is-more.

Contributors

Natalie Armstrong initially conceptualised and planned the Element, with input from Caroline Cupit and Carolyn Tarrant. Caroline Cupit wrote the first draft under Natalie Armstrong's supervision, with contributions from Natalie Armstrong and Carolyn Tarrant. All authors contributed to revising the Element in response to reviewer feedback. All authors have approved the final version.

Conflicts of Interest

None.

Acknowledgements

We thank the peer reviewers for their insightful comments and recommendations to improve the Element. A list of peer reviewers is published at www.cambridge.org/IQ-peer-reviewers.

Funding

This Element was funded by THIS Institute (The Healthcare Improvement Studies Institute, www.thisinstitute.cam.ac.uk). THIS Institute is strengthening the evidence base for improving the quality and safety of healthcare. THIS Institute is supported by a grant to the University of Cambridge from the Health Foundation – an independent charity committed to bringing about better health and healthcare for people in the UK.

Natalie Armstrong is supported by a Health Foundation Improvement Science Fellowship. Natalie Armstrong and Carolyn Tarrant are supported by the National Institute for Health Research (NIHR) Applied Research Collaboration East Midlands (ARC EM). The views expressed are those of the authors and not necessarily those of the NHS, the NIHR, or the Department of Health and Social Care. Caroline Cupit is supported by a Mildred Blaxter Fellowship from the Foundation for the Sociology of Health and Illness.

About the Authors

Caroline Cupit is a social scientist, working at the University of Leicester and the University of Oxford. She uses sociological theory and methods and has particular expertise in institutional ethnography – an approach she employs to identify good care practices as well as systems and processes for improvement.

Carolyn Tarrant is Professor of Health Services Research and leads the Social Science Applied to Healthcare Improvement Research (SAPPHIRE) Group at the University of Leicester. She is a social scientist with expertise in qualitative methods, including ethnographic methods in applied healthcare research.

Natalie Armstrong is Professor of Healthcare Improvement Research at the University of Leicester and Health Foundation Improvement Science Fellow. A medical sociologist by background, her work uses sociological ideas and methods to understand health and illness and to tackle problems in the delivery of high-quality healthcare.

Creative Commons Licence

References

1. Korenstein D, Falk R, Howell EA, Bishop T, Keyhani S. Overuse of health care services in the United States: an understudied problem. *Arch Intern Med* 2012; 172: 171–8. http://doi.org/10.1001/archinternmed.2011.772.

2. Nassery N, Segal JB, Chang E, Bridges JFP. Systematic overuse of health-care services: a conceptual model. *Appl Health Econ Health Policy* 2015; 13: 1–6. https://doi.org/10.1007/s40258-014-0126-5.

3. Organisation for Economic Co-operation and Development. *Tackling Wasteful Spending on Health*. Paris: OECD; 2017. www.oecd.org/health/tackling-wasteful-spending-on-health-9789264266414-en.htm (accessed 31 May 2022).

4. Saini V, Brownlee S, Elshaug AG, Glasziou P, Heath I. Addressing overuse and underuse around the world. *Lancet* 2017; 390: 105–7. https://doi.org/10.1016/S0140-6736(16)32573-9.

5. Berwick DM. Avoiding overuse – the next quality frontier. *Lancet* 2017; 390: 102–4. https://doi.org/10.1016/S0140-6736(16)32570-3.

6. Brownlee S, Chalkidou K, Doust J, et al. Evidence for overuse of medical services around the world. *Lancet* 2017; 390: 156–68. https://doi.org/10.1016/S0140-6736(16)32585-5.

7. Alderwick H, Robertson R, Appleby J, Dunn P, McGuire D. *Better Value in the NHS: the Role of Changes in Clinical Practice*. London: The King's Fund; 2015. www.kingsfund.org.uk/publications/better-value-nhs (accessed 31 May 2022).

8. Chassin MR, Galvin RW, National Roundtable on Health Care Quality. The urgent need to improve health care quality: Institute of Medicine national roundtable on health care quality. *JAMA* 1998; 280: 1000–5. https://doi.org/10.1001/jama.280.11.1000.

9. Moynihan R, Doust J, Henry D. Preventing overdiagnosis: how to stop harming the healthy. *BMJ* 2012; 344: e3502. http://dx.doi.org/10.1136/bmj.e3502.

10. Godlee F. Overtreatment, over here. *BMJ* 2012; 345: e6684. https://doi.org/10.1136/bmj.e6684.

11. Glasziou P, Moynihan R, Richards T, Godlee F. Too much medicine; too little care. *BMJ* 2013; 347: f4247. http://dx.doi.org/10.1136/bmj.f4247.

12. Carter SM, Rogers W, Heath I, et al. The challenge of overdiagnosis begins with its definition. *BMJ* 2015; 350: h869. https://dx.doi.org/10.1136/bmj.h869.

13. Brook RH, Chassin MR, Fink A, et al. A method for the detailed assessment of the appropriateness of medical technologies. *Int J Technol Assess Health Care* 1986; 2: 53–63. https://doi.org/10.1017/S0266462300002774.

14. Porter ME. What is value in health care? *N Engl J Med* 2010; 363: 2477–81. https://doi.org/10.1056/NEJMp1011024.

15. Baker DW, Qaseem A, Reynolds P, Gardner LA, Schneider EC. Design and use of performance measures to decrease low-value services and achieve cost-conscious care. *Ann Intern Med* 2013; 158: 55. https://doi.org/10.7326/0003-4819-158-1-201301010-00560.

16. Aylward M, Phillips C, Howson H. *Simply Prudent Healthcare – Achieving Better Care and Value for Money in Wales – Discussion Paper*. Swansea: Bevan Commission; 2013. www.bevancommission.org/publications/simply-prudent-healthcare-achieving-better-care-and-value-for-money-in-wales (accessed 31 May 2022).

17. MacLeod S, Musich S, Hawkins K, Schwebke K. Highlighting a common quality of care delivery problem: overuse of low-value healthcare services. *J Healthc Qual* 2018; 40: 201–8. https://doi.org/10.1097/JHQ.0000000000000095.

18. Hensher M, Tisdell J, Zimitat C. 'Too much medicine': insights and explanations from economic theory and research. *Soc Sci Med* 2017; 176: 77–84. https://doi.org/10.1016/j.socscimed.2017.01.020.

19. Lipitz-Snyderman A, Bach PB. Overuse of health care services: when less is more . . . more or less. *JAMA Intern Med* 2013; 173: 1277–8. https://doi.org/10.1001/jamainternmed.2013.6181.

20. Chan KS, Chang E, Nassery N, Chang H-Y, Segal JB. The state of overuse measurement: a critical review. *Med Care Res Rev* 2013; 70: 473–96. https://doi.org/10.1177/1077558713492202.

21. Verkerk EW, Tanke MAC, Kool RB, van Dulmen SA, Westert GP. Limit, lean or listen? A typology of low-value care that gives direction in de-implementation. *Int J Qual Health Care* 2018; 30: 736–9. https://doi.org/10.1093/intqhc/mzy100.

22. Elshaug AG, Watt AM, Mundy L, Willis CD. Over 150 potentially low-value health care practices: an Australian study. *Med J Aust* 2012; 197: 556–60. https://doi.org/10.5694/mja12.11083.

23. Robinson S, Williams I, Dickinson H, Freeman T, Rumbold B. Priority-setting and rationing in healthcare: evidence from the English experience. *Soc Sci Med* 2012; 75: 2386–93. https://doi.org/10.1016/j.socscimed.2012.09.014.

24. Macdonald H, Loder E. Too much medicine: the challenge of finding common ground. *BMJ* 2015; 350: h1163. https://doi.org/10.1136/bmj .h1163.

25. Garner S, Docherty M, Somner J, et al. Reducing ineffective practice: challenges in identifying low-value health care using Cochrane systematic reviews. *J Health Serv Res Policy* 2013; 18: 6–12. https://doi.org/10.1258/ jhsrp.2012.012044.

26. Altman DG, Bland JM. Absence of evidence is not evidence of absence. *BMJ* 1995; 311: 485. https://doi.org/10.1136/bmj.311.7003.485.

27. Verkerk EW, Huisman-de Waal G, Vermeulen H, et al. Low-value care in nursing: a systematic assessment of clinical practice guidelines. *Int J Nurs Stud* 2018; 87: 34–9. https://doi.org/10.1016/j.ijnurstu.2018.07.002.

28. Wieringa S, Dreesens D, Forland F, et al. Different knowledge, different styles of reasoning: a challenge for guideline development. *Br Med J Evid Based Med* 2018; 23: 87–91. http://dx.doi.org/10.1136/bmjebm-2017-110844.

29. Knaapen L. Being 'evidence-based' in the absence of evidence: the management of non-evidence in guideline development. *Soc Stud Sci* 2013; 43: 681–706. https://doi.org/10.1177/0306312713483679.

30. Keyhani S, Siu AL. The underuse of overuse research. *Health Serv Res* 2008; 43: 1923–30. https://doi.org/10.1111/j.1475-6773.2008.00920.x.

31. Shekelle P. The appropriateness method. *Med Decis Making* 2004; 24: 228–31. https://doi.org/10.1177/0272989X04264212.

32. Keyhani S, Falk R, Howell EA, Bishop T, Korenstein D. Overuse and systems of care: a systematic review. *Med Care* 2013; 51: 503–8. https:// doi.org/10.1097/MLR.0b013e31828dbafe.

33. Garner S, Littlejohns P. Disinvestment from low value clinical interventions: NICEly done? *BMJ* 2011; 343: d4519. https://doi.org/10.1136/bmj .d4519.

34. National Institute for Health and Care Excellence. Cut NHS waste through NICE's 'do not do' database. NICE; 6 November 2014. www.nice.org.uk/ news/article/cut-nhs-waste-through-nice-s–do-not-do–database (accessed 16 May 2019).

35. Polisena J, Clifford T, Elshaug AG, et al. Case studies that illustrate disinvestment and resource allocation decision-making processes in health care: a systematic review. *Int J Technol Assess Health Care* 2013; 29: 174–84. https://doi.org/10.1017/S0266462313000068.

36. Noseworthy T, Clement F. Health technology reassessment: scope, methodology, & language. *Int J Technol Assess Health Care* 2012; 28: 201–2. https://doi.org/10.1017/S0266462312000359.

37. Sevick K, Soril LJJ, MacKean G, Noseworthy TW, Clement FM. Unpacking early experiences with health technology reassessment in a complex healthcare system. *Int J Healthcare Manage* 2020; 13: 156–62. https://doi.org/10.1080/20479700.2017.1337679.

38. Soril LJJ, Niven DJ, Esmail R, Noseworthy TW, Clement FM. Untangling, unbundling, and moving forward: framing health technology reassessment in the changing conceptual landscape. *Int J Technol Assess Health Care* 2018; 34: 212–7. https://doi.org/10.1017/S0266462318000120.

39. Leape LL, Park RE, Solomon DH, et al. Does inappropriate use explain small-area variations in the use of health care services? *JAMA* 1990; 263: 669–72. https://doi.org/10.1001/jama.1990.03440050063034.

40. Chen CL, Lin GA, Bardach NS, et al. Preoperative medical testing in Medicare patients undergoing cataract surgery. *N Engl J Med*. 2015; 372: 1530–8. https://doi.org/10.1056/NEJMsa1410846.

41. Organisation for Economic Co-operation and Development. *Geographic Variations in Health Care: What Do We Know and What Can Be Done to Improve Health System Performance?* Paris: OECD; 2014. www.oecd.org/health/geographic-variations-in-health-care-9789264216594-en.htm (accessed 31 May 2022).

42. Public Health England. *The NHS Atlas of Variation in Healthcare: Reducing Unwarranted Variation to Increase Value and Improve Quality. September 2016*. London: Public Health England; 2015. https://fingertips.phe.org.uk/documents/atlas_2015%20compendium.pdf (accessed 31 May 2022).

43. Wennberg JE, Barnes BA, Zubkoff M. Professional uncertainty and the problem of supplier-induced demand. *Soc Sci Med* 1982; 16: 811–24. https://doi.org/10.1016/0277-9536(82)90234-9.

44. Schang L, Morton A, DaSilva P, Bevan G. From data to decisions? Exploring how healthcare payers respond to the NHS Atlas of Variation in Healthcare in England. *Health Policy* 2014; 114: 79–87. https://doi.org/10.1016/j.healthpol.2013.04.014.

45. Australian Commission on Safety and Quality in Healthcare. *Exploring Healthcare Variation in Australia: Analyses Resulting from an OECD Study*. Sydney: ACSQHC; 2014. www.safetyandquality.gov.au/publications-and-resources/resource-library/exploring-healthcare-variation-australia-analyses-resulting-oecd-study (accessed 31 May 2022).

46. Public Health England. AMR local indicators. Published 15 October 2020. https://fingertips.phe.org.uk/profile/amr-local-indicators (accessed 31 May 2022).

47. European Centre for Disease Prevention and Control. *Antimicrobial Consumption in the EU/EEA (ESAC-Net) – Annual Epidemiological Report 2020*. ECDPC; 2021. www.ecdc.europa.eu/en/publications-data/ surveillance-antimicrobial-consumption-europe-2020 (accessed 31 May 2022).

48. Levinson W, Kallewaard M, Bhatia RS, et al. 'Choosing Wisely': a growing international campaign. *BMJ Qual Saf* 2015; 24: 167–74. https://doi.org/10.1136/bmjqs-2014-003821.

49. Schwartz AL, Landon BE, Elshaug AG, Chernew ME, McWilliams JM. Measuring low-value care in Medicare. *JAMA Intern Med* 2014; 174: 1067–76. https://doi.org/10.1001/jamainternmed.2014.1541.

50. Segal JB, Bridges JF, Chang H-Y, et al. Identifying possible indicators of systematic overuse of health care procedures with claims data. *Med Care* 2014; 52: 157–63. https://doi.org/10.1097/MLR.0000000000000052.

51. Chalmers K, Badgery-Parker T, Pearson S-A, et al. Developing indicators for measuring low-value care: mapping Choosing Wisely recommendations to hospital data. *BMC Res Notes* 2018; 11: 163. https://doi.org/ 10.1186/s13104-018-3270-4.

52. Isaac T, Rosenthal MB, Colla CH, et al. Measuring overuse with electronic health records data. *Am J Manag Care* 2018; 24: 19–25. www.ajmc.com/ view/measuring-overuse-with-electronic-health-records-data (accessed 31 May 2022).

53. Brett J, Elshaug AG, Bhatia RS, et al. A methodological protocol for selecting and quantifying low-value prescribing practices in routinely collected data: an Australian case study. *Implement Sci* 2017; 12: 58. https://doi.org/10.1186/s13012-017-0585-9.

54. Haynes RB, Devereaux PJ, Guyatt GH. Clinical expertise in the era of evidence-based medicine and patient choice. *Evid Based Med* 2002; 7: 36–8. https://doi.org/10.1136/ebm.7.2.36.

55. National Institute for Health and Care Excellence. Assessing cost effectiveness. In: NICE. *The Guidelines Manual: Process and Methods*. London: NICE; 2012: chapter 7. www.nice.org.uk/process/pmg6/chapter/assessing-cost-effectiveness (accessed 8 May 2018).

56. Upshur R. Looking for rules in a world of exceptions: reflections on evidence-based practice. *Perspect Biol Med* 2005; 48: 477–89. https:// doi.org/10.1353/pbm.2005.0098.

57. Timmermans S, Berg M. *The Gold Standard: The Challenge of Evidence-Based Medicine and Standardization in Health Care*. Philadelphia, PA: Temple University Press; 2010.

58. Mykhalovskiy E, Weir L. The problem of evidence-based medicine: directions for social science. *Soc Sci Med* 2004; 59: 1059–69. https://doi.org/10.1016/j.socscimed.2003.12.002.

59. Greenhalgh T, Howick J, Maskrey N. Evidence based medicine: a movement in crisis? *BMJ* 2014; 348: g3725. https://doi.org/10.1136/bmj.g3725.

60. Knaapen L. Evidence-based medicine or cookbook medicine? Addressing concerns over the standardization of care. *Sociol Compass* 2014; 8: 823–36. https://doi.org/10.1111/soc4.12184.

61. Williams I, Brown H. *Factors Influencing Decisions of Value in Health Care: a Review of the Literature*. Birmingham: Health Service Management Centre, University of Birmingham; 2014.

62. Williams I, Harlock J, Robert G, et al. Decommissioning health care: identifying best practice through primary and secondary research – a prospective mixed-methods study. *Health Serv Deliv Res* 2017; 5: 22. https://doi.org/10.3310/hsdr05220.

63. Malik HT, Marti J, Darzi A, Mossialos E. Savings from reducing low-value general surgical interventions. *Br J Surg* 2018; 105: 13–25. https://doi.org/10.1002/bjs.10719.

64. Tarrant C, Krockow EM, Nakkawita WMID, et al. Moral and contextual dimensions of 'inappropriate' antibiotic prescribing in secondary care: a three-country interview study. *Front Sociol* 2020; 5: 7. https://doi.org/10.3389/fsoc.2020.00007.

65. Dyar OJ, Obua C, Chandy S, et al. Using antibiotics responsibly: are we there yet? *Future Microbiol* 2016; 11: 1057–71. https://doi.org/10.2217/fmb-2016-0041.

66. Korenstein D. Patient perception of benefits and harms: the Achilles heel of high-value care. *JAMA Intern Med* 2015; 175: 287–8. https://doi.org/10.1001/jamainternmed.2014.6744.

67. Hollon SD, Areán PA, Craske MG, et al. Development of clinical practice guidelines. *Ann Rev Clin Psychol* 2014; 10: 213–41. https://doi.org/10.1146/annurev-clinpsy-050212-185529.

68. Heneghan C, Mahtani KR, Goldacre B, et al. Evidence based medicine manifesto for better healthcare. *BMJ* 2017; 357: j2973. https://doi.org/10.1136/bmj.j2973.

69. Pathak EB, Wieten S, Djulbegovic B. Critical reflections on value in medicine. *J Med Pers* 2013; 11: 69–72. https://doi.org/10.1007/s12682-013-0153-2.

70. Gøtzsche PC, Jørgensen KJ. Screening for breast cancer with mammography. *Cochrane Database Syst Rev* 2013; 6: CD001877. https://doi.org/10.1002/14651858.CD001877.pub5.

71. Independent UK Panel on Breast Cancer Screening. The benefits and harms of breast cancer screening: an independent review. *Lancet* 2012; 380: 1778–86. https://doi.org/10.1016/S0140-6736(12)61611-0.

72. Hersch J, Barratt A, Jansen J, et al. Use of a decision aid including information on overdetection to support informed choice about breast cancer screening: a randomised controlled trial. *Lancet* 2015; 385: 1642–52. https://doi.org/10.1016/S0140-6736(15)60123-4.

73. Stiggelbout A, Copp T, Jacklyn G, et al. Women's acceptance of over-detection in breast cancer screening: can we assess harm-benefit tradeoffs? *Med Decis Making* 2020; 40: 42–51. https://doi.org/10.1177/0272989X19 886886.

74. Stacey D, Légaré F, Col NF, et al. Decision aids for people facing health treatment or screening decisions. *Cochrane Database Syst Rev* 2014; 1: CD001431. https://doi.org/10.1002/14651858.CD001431.pub4.

75. Morden NE, Colla CH, Sequist TD, Rosenthal MB. Choosing Wisely – the politics and economics of labeling low-value services. *N Engl J Med* 2014; 370: 589–92. https://doi.org/10.1056/NEJMp1314965.

76. Hasson H, Nilsen P, Augustsson H, et al. To do or not to do – balancing governance and professional autonomy to abandon low-value practices: a study protocol. *Implement Sci* 2019; 14: 70. https://doi.org/10.1186/s13012-019-0919-x

77. National Institute for Health and Care Excellence. *Cardiovascular Disease: Risk Assessment and Reduction, Including Lipid Modification. Clinical Guideline.* London: NICE; 2014. www.nice.org.uk/guidance/CG181 (accessed 31 May 2022).

78. Gallagher J. Statins: millions more to get drugs in controversial plans. *BBC News*; 18 July 2014. www.bbc.co.uk/news/health-28352290 (accessed 10 May 2015).

79. Public Health England. *Action on Cardiovascular Disease: Getting Serious About Prevention.* London: PHE; 2016. https://tinyurl.com/y4ehujwk (accessed 31 October 2015).

80. NHS Health Check. Reducing heart attack and stroke: STP level size of the prize infographic and NHS health check factsheet. www.healthcheck.nhs .uk/commissioners-and-providers/data/size-of-the-prize-and-nhs-health-check-factsheet (accessed 31 May 2022).

81. NHS Digital. Quality and Outcomes Framework. Leeds: NHS Digital; 2017. https://webarchive.nationalarchives.gov.uk/ukgwa/20180328132022/https://digital.nhs.uk/article/8910/Quality-and-Outcome-Framework-QOF-Indicators-No-Longer-In-QOF-INLIQ-Enhanced-Services-ES-

Vaccinations-and-Immunisations-V-I-and-GMS-Core-Contract-CC-extrac
tion-specifications-business-rules- (accessed 16 November 2022).

82. Montori VM, Brito JP, Ting HH. Patient-centered and practical application of new high cholesterol guidelines to prevent cardiovascular disease. *JAMA* 2014; 311: 465–6. https://doi.org/10.1001/jama.2014.110.

83. Heath I. Role of fear in overdiagnosis and overtreatment – an essay by Iona Heath. *BMJ* 2014; 349: g6123. https://doi.org/10.1136/bmj.g6123.

84. Hutchins R, Viera AJ, Sheridan SL, Pignone MP. Quantifying the utility of taking pills for cardiovascular prevention. *Circ Cardiovasc Qual Outcomes* 2015; 8: 155–63. https://doi.org/10.1161/CIRCOUTCOMES .114.001240.

85. Husten L. The Lancet versus BMJ: dispatch from the statin wars. *CardioBrief*, 15 September 2016. http://cardiobrief.org/2016/09/15/the-lancet-versus-bmj-dispatch-from-the-statin-wars (accessed 26 September 2016).

86. Kendrick M. Are statins overused? *Future Lipidol* 2007; 2: 481–3. https:// doi.org/10.2217/17460875.2.5.481.

87. Newman DH, Redberg RF. Will new statin guidelines lead to overtreatment? *Clin Lipidol* 2014; 9: 125–8. https://doi.org/10.2217/ clp.14.9.

88. Capewell S, McCartney M, Holland W. Invited debate: NHS health checks – a naked emperor? *J Public Health* 2015; 37: 187–92. https://doi .org/10.1093/pubmed/fdv063.

89. Mafi JN, Parchman M. Low-value care: an intractable global problem with no quick fix. *BMJ Qual Saf* 2018; 27: 333–6. https://doi.org/10.1136/ bmjqs-2017-007477.

90. Academy of Royal Medical Colleges. *Protecting Resources, Promoting Value: A Doctor's Guide to Cutting Waste in Clinical Care*. London: AoMRC; 2014. www.aomrc.org.uk/reports-guidance/protecting-resources-promoting-value-1114 (accessed 14 January 2020).

91. Ellen ME, Wilson MG, Vélez M, et al. Addressing overuse of health services in health systems: a critical interpretive synthesis. *Health Res Policy Syst* 2018; 16: 48. https://doi.org/10.1186/s12961-018-0325-x.

92. Saini V, Garcia-Armesto S, Klemperer D, et al. Drivers of poor medical care. *Lancet* 2017; 390: 178–90. https://doi.org/10.1016/S0140-6736(16) 30947-3.

93. Kleinert S, Horton R. From universal health coverage to right care for health. *Lancet* 2017; 390: 101–2. https://doi.org/10.1016/S0140-6736(16) 32588-0.

94. Glasziou P, Straus S, Brownlee S, et al. Evidence for underuse of effective medical services around the world. *Lancet* 2017; 390: 169–77. https://doi.org/10.1016/S0140-6736(16)30946-1.

95. Elshaug AG, Rosenthal MB, Lavis JN, et al. Levers for addressing medical underuse and overuse: achieving high-value health care. *Lancet* 2017; 390: 191–202. https://doi.org/10.1016/S0140-6736(16)32586-7.

96. Jain A. Too much medicine is not just a problem of rich countries. *BMJ* 2015; 350: h1095. https://doi.org/10.1136/bmj.h1095.

97. Willis LD, Chandler C. Quick fix for care, productivity, hygiene and inequality: reframing the entrenched problem of antibiotic overuse. *BMJ Global Health* 2019; 4: e001590. http://dx.doi.org/10.1136/bmjgh-2019-001590.

98. Hicks LK. Reframing overuse in health care: time to focus on the harms. *J Oncol Pract* 2015; 11: 168–70. https://doi.org/10.1200/JOP.2015.004283.

99. Norton WE, Kennedy AE, Chambers DA. Studying de-implementation in health: an analysis of funded research grants. *Implement Sci* 2017; 12: 144. https://doi.org/10.1186/s13012-017-0655-z.

100. Moriates C. Overuse as a patient safety problem. *Patient Safety Network*; 1 September 2014. http://psnet.ahrq.gov/perspective/overuse-patient-safety-problem (accessed 10 April 2020).

101. Berwick DM, Hackbarth AD. Eliminating waste in US health care. *JAMA* 2012; 307: 1513–16. https://doi.org/10.1001/jama.2012.362.

102. Institute for Healthcare Improvement. Across the chasm: six aims for changing the health care system. *IHI*; undated. www.ihi.org:80/resources/Pages/ImprovementStories/AcrosstheChasmSixAimsforChangingtheHealthCareSystem.aspx (31 May 2022).

103. Armstrong N. Overdiagnosis and overtreatment as a quality problem: insights from healthcare improvement research. *BMJ Qual Saf* 2018; 27: 571–5. http://dx.doi.org/10.1136/bmjqs-2017-007571.

104. Lipitz-Snyderman A, Korenstein D. Reducing overuse – is patient safety the answer? *JAMA* 2017; 317: 810–1. https://doi.org/10.1001/jama.2017.0896.

105. Pathirana T, Clark J, Moynihan R. Mapping the drivers of overdiagnosis to potential solutions. *BMJ* 2017; 358: j3879. https://doi.org/10.1136/bmj.j3879.

106. Richardson J, Peacock S. *Reconsidering Theories and Evidence of Supplier Induced Cemand*. Melbourne: Centre for Health Economics, Monash University; 2006. https://bridges.monash.edu/articles/journal_contribution/Reconsidering_theories_and_evidence_of_supplier_induced_demand/5090458 (accessed 31 May 2022).

107. Siemieniuk RAC, Harris IA, Agoritsas T, et al. Arthroscopic surgery for degenerative knee arthritis and meniscal tears: a clinical practice guideline. *BMJ* 2017; 357: j1982. https://doi.org/10.1136/bmj.j1982.

108. Armstrong N, Hilton P. Doing diagnosis: whether and how clinicians use a diagnostic tool of uncertain clinical utility. *Social Sci Med* 2014; 120: 208–14. https://doi.org/10.1016/j.socscimed.2014.09.032.

109. Lyu H, Xu T, Brotman D, et al. Overtreatment in the United States. *PLoS One* 2017; 12: e0181970. https://doi.org/10.1371/journal.pone.0181970.

110. Mulley AG. Inconvenient truths about supplier induced demand and unwarranted variation in medical practice. *BMJ* 2009; 339: b4073. https://doi.org/10.1136/bmj.b4073

111. Stamatakis E, Weiler R, Ioannidis JPA. Undue industry influences that distort healthcare research, strategy, expenditure and practice: a review. *Eur J Clin Invest* 2013; 43: 469–75. https://doi.org/10.1111/eci.12074.

112. Prasad V, Vandross A, Toomey C, et al. A decade of reversal: an analysis of 146 contradicted medical practices. *Mayo Clin Proc* 2013; 88: 790–8. https://doi.org/10.1016/j.mayocp.2013.05.012.

113. Moynihan R, Smith R. Too much medicine? *BMJ* 2002; 324: 859. https://doi.org/10.1136/bmj.324.7342.859.

114. Fleck F. Realistic medicine to improve the quality of care in Scotland. *Bull World Health Organ* 2016; 95: 395–6. https://doi.org/10.2471/BLT.17.030617.

115. ABIM Foundation. Choosing Wisely. https://abimfoundation.org/what-we-do/choosing-wisely (accessed 15 May 2019).

116. Malhotra A, Maughan D, Ansell J, et al. Choosing Wisely in the UK: the Academy of Medical Royal Colleges' initiative to reduce the harms of too much medicine. *BMJ* 2015; 350: h2308. https://doi.org/10.1136/bmj.h2308.

117. Torjesen I. Royal colleges issue list of 40 unnecessary interventions. *BMJ* 2016; 355: i5732. https://doi.org/10.1136/bmj.i5732.

118. Welsh Government. *Prudent Healthcare: Securing Health and Well-Being for Future Generations*. Cardiff: Welsh Government; 2016. https://gov.wales/sites/default/files/publications/2019-04/securing-health-and-well-being-for-future-generations.pdf (accessed 5 April 2020).

119. Fenning SJ, Smith G, Calderwood C. Realistic Medicine: changing culture and practice in the delivery of health and social care. *Patient Educ Couns* 2019; 102: 1751–5. https://doi.org/10.1016/j.pec.2019.06.024.

120. Scott IA, Duckett SJ. In search of professional consensus in defining and reducing low-value care. *Med J Aust* 2015; 203: 179–81. https://doi.org/10.5694/mja14.01664.

121. Horvath K, Semlitsch T, Jeitler K, et al. Choosing Wisely: assessment of current US top five list recommendations' trustworthiness using a pragmatic approach. *BMJ Open* 2016; 6: e012366. http://dx.doi.org/10.1136/bmjopen-2016-012366.

122. Colla CH, Morden NE, Sequist TD, Schpero WL, Rosenthal MB. Choosing Wisely: prevalence and correlates of low-value health care services in the United States. *J Gen Intern Med* 2015; 30: 221–8. https://doi.org/10.1007/s11606-014-3070-z.

123. Wolfson D, Santa J, Slass L. Engaging physicians and consumers in conversations about treatment overuse and waste: a short history of the Choosing Wisely campaign. *Acad Med* 2014; 89: 990–5. https://doi.org/10.1097/ACM.0000000000000270.

124. Rosenberg A, Agiro A, Gottlieb M, et al. Early trends among seven recommendations from the Choosing Wisely campaign. *JAMA Intern Med* 2015; 175: 1913–20. https://doi.org/10.1001/jamainternmed.2015.5441.

125. Hong AS, Ross-Degnan D, Zhang F, Wharam JF. Small decline in low-value back imaging associated with the 'Choosing Wisely' campaign, 2012-14. *Health Aff* 2017; 36: 671–9. https://doi.org/10.1377/hlthaff.2016.1263.

126. Bhatia RS, Levinson W, Shortt S, et al. Measuring the effect of Choosing Wisely: an integrated framework to assess campaign impact on low-value care. *BMJ Qual Saf* 2015; 24: 523–31. http://dx.doi.org/10.1136/bmjqs-2015-004070.

127. McCartney M, Treadwell J. The RCGP's new standing group on over-diagnosis. *BMJ* 2014; 349: g4454. https://doi.org/10.1136/bmj.g4454.

128. Parkinson B, Sermet C, Clement F, et al. Disinvestment and value-based purchasing strategies for pharmaceuticals: an international review. *PharmacoEcon* 2015; 33: 905–24. https://doi.org/10.1007/s40273-015-0293-8.

129. Niven DJ, Mrklas KJ, Holodinsky JK, et al. Towards understanding the de-adoption of low-value clinical practices: a scoping review. *BMC Med* 2015; 13: 255. https://doi.org/10.1186/s12916-015-0488-z.

130. Parker G, Rappon T, Berta W. Active change interventions to de-implement low-value healthcare practices: a scoping review protocol. *BMJ Open* 2019; 9: e027370. https://doi.org/10.1136/bmjopen-2018-027370.

131. MacKean G, Noseworthy T, Elshaug AG, et al. Health technology reassessment: the art of the possible. *Int J Technol Assess Health Care* 2013; 29: 418–23. https://doi.org/10.1017/S0266462313000494.

132. Wammes JJG, van den Akker-van Marle ME, Verkerk EW, et al. Identifying and prioritizing lower value services from Dutch specialist guidelines and a comparison with the UK do-not-do list. *BMC Med* 2016; 14: 196. https://doi.org/10.1186/s12916-016-0747-7.

133. Colla CH, Mainor AJ, Hargreaves C, Sequist T, Morden N. Interventions aimed at reducing use of low-value health services: a systematic review. *Med Care Res Rev* 2017; 74: 507–50. https://doi.org/10.1177/1077558716656970.

134. Radnor Z, Williams S. Lean and associated techniques for process improvement. In: Dixon-Woods M, Brown K, Marjanovic S, et al., editors. *Elements of Improving Quality and Safety in Healthcare*. Cambridge: Cambridge University Press; forthcoming.

135. Tannenbaum C, Martin P, Tamblyn R, Benedetti A, Ahmed S. Reduction of inappropriate benzodiazepine prescriptions among older adults through direct patient education: the EMPOWER cluster randomized trial. *JAMA Intern Med* 2014; 174: 890–8. https://doi.org/10.1001/jamainternmed.2014.949.

136. Chen HY, Harris IA, Sutherland K, Levesque J-F. A controlled before-after study to evaluate the effect of a clinician led policy to reduce knee arthroscopy in NSW. *BMC Musculoskelet Disord* 2018; 19: 148. https://doi.org/10.1186/s12891-018-2043-5.

137. McCaffery KJ, Jansen J, Scherer LD, et al. Walking the tightrope: communicating overdiagnosis in modern healthcare. *BMJ* 2016; 352: i348. https://doi.org/10.1136/bmj.i348.

138. Morgan DJ, Leppin A, Smith CD, Korenstein D. A practical framework for understanding and reducing medical overuse: conceptualizing overuse through the patient-clinician interaction. *J Hosp Med* 2017; 12: 346–51. https://doi.org/10.12788/jhm.2738.

139. The Health Foundation. *The MAGIC Programme: Evaluation*. London: The Health Foundation; 2013. www.health.org.uk/publications/the-magic-programme-evaluation (accessed 31 May 2022).

140. Coulter A. *Implementing Shared Decision Making in the UK*. London: The Health Foundation; 2010. www.health.org.uk/publications/implementing-shared-decision-making-in-the-uk (accessed 31 May 2022).

141. Stacey D, Légaré F, Lewis K, et al. Decision aids for people facing health treatment or screening decisions. *Cochrane Database Syst Rev* 2017; 4: CD001431. https://doi.org/10.1002/14651858.CD001431.pub5.

142. Joseph-Williams N, Lloyd A, Edwards A, et al. Implementing shared decision making in the NHS: lessons from the MAGIC programme. *BMJ* 2017; 357: j1744. https://doi.org/10.1136/bmj.j1744.

143. Duerden M, Avery T, Payne R. *Polypharmacy and Medicines Optimisation: Making It Safe and Sound.* London: The King's Fund; 2013. www.kingsfund.org.uk/publications/polypharmacy-and-medicines-optimisation (accessed 31 May 2022).

144. NHS England. *Medicines Optimisation in Care Homes: Programme Overview.* NHS England; 2018. www.england.nhs.uk/publication/medicines-optimisation-in-care-homes-programme-overview (accessed 31 May 2022).

145. Alves A, Green S, James DH. Deprescribing of medicines in care homes – a five-year evaluation of primary care pharmacist practices. *Pharmacy* 2019; 7: 105. https://doi.org/10.3390/pharmacy7030105.

146. Reeve E, Bell JS, Hilmer SN. Barriers to optimising prescribing and deprescribing in older adults with dementia: a narrative review. *Curr Clin Pharmacol* 2015; 10: 168–77. https://doi.org/10.2174/157488471003150820150330.

147. The Health Foundation. Pills: reviewing medication in care homes. www.health.org.uk/news-and-comment/featured-content/power-of-people/pills (accessed 31 May 2022).

148. Maratt JK, Kerr EA, Klamerus ML, et al. Measures used to assess the impact of interventions to reduce low-value care: a systematic review. *J Gen Intern Med* 2019; 34: 1857–64. https://doi.org/10.1007/s11606-019-05069-5.

149. Van Dijck C, Vlieghe E, Cox JA. Antibiotic stewardship interventions in hospitals in low-and middle-income countries: a systematic review. *Bull World Health Organ* 2018; 96: 266–80. www.ncbi.nlm.nih.gov/pmc/articles/PMC5872012/ (accessed 31 May 2022).

150. Wilson P, Kislov R. Implementation science. In: Dixon-Woods M, Brown K, Marjanovic S, et al., editors. *Elements of Improving Quality and Safety in Healthcare.* Cambridge: Cambridge University Press; 2022. https://doi.org/10.1017/9781009237055.

151. Oakes AH, Chang H-Y, Segal JB. Systemic overuse of health care in a commercially insured US population, 2010-2015. *BMC Health Serv Res* 2019; 19: 280. https://doi.org/10.1186/s12913-019-4079-0.

152. King R. What not to do. *InSight+*; 15 September 2014. https://insightplus.mja.com.au/2014/34/richard-king-what-not-do (accessed 7 September 2020).

153. de Vries EF, Struijs JN, Heijink R, Hendrikx RJP, Baan CA. Are low-value care measures up to the task? A systematic review of the literature. *BMC Health Serv Res* 2016; 16: 405. https://doi.org/10.1186/s12913-016-1656-3.

154. Harvey G, McInnes E. Disinvesting in ineffective and inappropriate practice: the neglected side of evidence-based health care? *Worldviews Evid Based Nurs* 2015; 12: 309–12. https://doi.org/10.1111/wvn.12137.

155. Williams I, Robinson S, Dickinson H. *Rationing in Health Care: the Theory and Practice of Priority Setting*. Bristol: Policy Press; 2012.

156. Hollingworth W, Rooshenas L, Busby J, et al. Using clinical practice variations as a method for commissioners and clinicians to identify and prioritise opportunities for disinvestment in health care: a cross-sectional study, systematic reviews and qualitative study. *Health Serv Deliv Res* 2015; 3: 13. https://doi.org/10.3310/hsdr03130.

157. Wye L, Brangan E, Cameron A, et al. Evidence based policy making and the 'art' of commissioning – how English healthcare commissioners access and use information and academic research in 'real life' decision-making: an empirical qualitative study. *BMC Health Serv Res* 2015; 15: 430. https://doi.org/10.1186/s12913-015-1091-x.

158. The Health Foundation. *Quality Improvement Made Simple*. London: The Health Foundation; 2021. www.health.org.uk/publications/quality-improvement-made-simple (accessed 31 May 2022).

159. Chassin MR. Improving the quality of health care: what's taking so long? *Health Aff* 2013; 32: 1761–5. https://doi.org/10.1377/hlthaff.2013.0809.

160. Parker G, Shahid N, Berta W. The use of theories and frameworks to understand and address the reduction of low-value healthcare practices: a scoping review. *BMJ Evid Based Med* 2018; 23: A51–A52. http://dx.doi.org/10.1136/bmjebm-2018-111070.109.

161. O'Keeffe M, Traeger AC, Hoffmann T, et al. Can nudge-interventions address health service overuse and underuse? Protocol for a systematic review. *BMJ Open* 2019; 9: e029540. https://doi.org/10.1136/bmjopen-2019-029540.

162. Owen-Smith A, Coast J, Donovan J. 'I can see where they're coming from, but when you're on the end of it . . . you just want to get the money and the drug.': explaining reactions to explicit healthcare rationing. *Soc Sci Med* 2009; 68: 1935–42. https://doi.org/10.1016/j.socscimed.2009.03.024.

163. Owen-Smith A, Coast J, Donovan J. The desirability of being open about health care rationing decisions: findings from a qualitative study of patients and clinical professionals. *J Health Serv Res Policy* 2010; 15: 14–20. https://doi.org/10.1258/jhsrp.2009.009045.

164. Hollingworth W, Rooshenas L, Busby J, et al. Using clinical practice variations as a method for commissioners and clinicians to identify and prioritise opportunities for disinvestment in health care: a cross-sectional

study, systematic reviews and qualitative study. *Health Serv Deliv Res* 2015; 3: 13, pp 55–85. https://doi.org/10.3310/hsdr03130.

165. NHS England. Evidence-based interventions programme. www.england .nhs.uk/evidence-based-interventions (accessed 11 March 2020).

166. NHS England, NHS Clinical Commissioners, Academy of Medical Royal Colleges, NHS Improvement, National Institute for Health and Care Excellence. *Evidence-Based Interventions: Guidance for CCGs*. Leeds: NHS England; 2018. www.aomrc.org.uk/ebi/wp-content/uploads/2021/ 05/ebi-statutory-guidance.pdf (accessed 31 May 2022).

167. Academy of Medical Royal Colleges. Evidence-based interventions. www.aomrc.org.uk/ebi/about (accessed 31 May 2022).

168. NHS England. Items which should not be routinely prescribed in primary care. www.england.nhs.uk/medicines/items-which-should-not-be-routinely-prescribed (accessed 8 September 2019).

169. NHS England. Frequently asked questions about evidence-based interventions. www.england.nhs.uk/coronavirus/secondary-care/other-resources/clinical-prioritisation-programme/clinical-prioritisation-pro gramme-frequently-asked-questions/frequently-asked-questions-about-evidence-based-interventions (accessed 31 May 2022).

170. Puntis J. *17 Evidence Based Interventions (17 EBI) – Where Are We Now? Campaigning over Treatment Access Policies*. London: Keep Our NHS Public; 2019. https://keepournhspublic.com/wp-content/uploads/2019/ 07/17-EBI-and-rationing-final.pdf (accessed 31 May 2022).

171. Wathen S. National Institute for Clinical Excellence (NICE) guidance ignored: NHS England rationing plan is not Nice at all. *Keep Our NHS Public*; 28 September 2018. https://keepournhspublic.com/national-institute-for-clinical-excellence-nice-guidance-ignored-nhs-england-rationing-plan-is-not-nice-at-all (accessed 31 May 2022).

172. Pulse News. GPs demand awareness campaign to explain new rationing scheme to patients. Pulse Today. *Pulse*; 18 December 2018. www.pulseto day.co.uk/news/referrals/gps-demand-awareness-campaign-to-explain-new-rationing-scheme-to-patients (accessed 31 May 2022).

173. Pandya A. Adding cost-effectiveness to define low-value care. *JAMA* 2018; 319: 1977–8. https://doi.org/10.1001/jama.2018.2856.

174. Tsevat J, Moriates C. Value-based health care meets cost-effectiveness analysis. *Ann Intern Med* 2018; 5: 329–32. https://doi.org/10.7326/M18-0342.

175. Bevan G, Brown LD. The political economy of rationing health care in England and the US: the 'accidental logics' of political settlements. *Health Econ Policy Law* 2014; 9: 273–94. https://doi.org/10.1017/ S1744133114000127.

176. Rooshenas L, Owen-Smith A, Hollingworth W, et al. 'I won't call it rationing ... ': an ethnographic study of healthcare disinvestment in theory and practice. *Soc Sci Med* 2015; 128: 273–81. https://doi.org/10.1016/j.socscimed.2015.01.020.

177. Ford A. The concept of exceptionality: a legal farce? *Med Law Rev* 2012; 20: 304–36. https://doi.org/10.1093/medlaw/fws002.

178. Russell J, Swinglehurst D, Greenhalgh T. 'Cosmetic boob jobs' or evidence-based breast surgery: an interpretive policy analysis of the rationing of 'low value' treatments in the English National Health Service. *BMC Health Serv Res* 2014; 14: 413. https://doi.org/10.1186/1472-6963-14-413.

179. Russell J, Greenhalgh T. Being 'rational' and being 'human': how National Health Service rationing decisions are constructed as rational by resource allocation panels. *Health* 2014; 18: 441–57. https://doi.org/10.1177/1363459313507586.

180. Heale W, Syrett K. Challenging NHS England's individual funding request policy. *British J Healthc Manag* 2018; 24: 218–21. https://doi.org/10.12968/bjhc.2018.24.5.218.

181. Hodgetts K, Elshaug AG, Hiller JE. What counts and how to count it: physicians' constructions of evidence in a disinvestment context. *Soc Sci Med* 2012; 75: 2191–9. https://doi.org/10.1016/j.socscimed.2012.08.016.

182. Entwistle V, Calnan M, Dieppe P. Consumer involvement in setting the health services research agenda: persistent questions of value. *J Health Serv Res Policy* 2008; 13: 76–81. https://doi.org/10.1258/jhsrp.2008.007167.

183. Cupit C, Armstrong N. A win-win scenario? Restrictive policies from alternative standpoints. *J Health Organ Manage* 2021; 35: 378–84. https://doi.org/10.1108/JHOM-06-2021-0239.

184. Hofmann B. Diagnosing overdiagnosis: conceptual challenges and suggested solutions. *Eur J Epidemiol* 2014; 29: 599–604. https://doi.org/10.1007/s10654-014-9920-5.

185. Cupit C, Rankin J, Armstrong N, Martin GP. Overruling uncertainty about preventative medications: the social organisation of healthcare professionals' knowledge and practices. *Sociol Health Illn* 2019; 42: 114–29. https://doi.org/10.1111/1467-9566.12998.

Cambridge Elements ≡

Improving Quality and Safety in Healthcare

Editors-in-Chief

Mary Dixon-Woods

THIS Institute (The Healthcare Improvement Studies Institute)

Mary is Director of THIS Institute and is the Health Foundation Professor of Healthcare Improvement Studies in the Department of Public Health and Primary Care at the University of Cambridge. Mary leads a programme of research focused on healthcare improvement, healthcare ethics, and methodological innovation in studying healthcare.

Graham Martin

THIS Institute (The Healthcare Improvement Studies Institute)

Graham is Director of Research at THIS Institute, leading applied research programmes and contributing to the institute's strategy and development. His research interests are in the organisation and delivery of healthcare, and particularly the role of professionals, managers, and patients and the public in efforts at organisational change.

Executive Editor

Katrina Brown

THIS Institute (The Healthcare Improvement Studies Institute)

Katrina is Communications Manager at THIS Institute, providing editorial expertise to maximise the impact of THIS Institute's research findings. She managed the project to produce the series.

Editorial Team

Sonja Marjanovic

RAND Europe

Sonja is Director of RAND Europe's healthcare innovation, industry, and policy research. Her work provides decision-makers with evidence and insights to support innovation and improvement in healthcare systems, and to support the translation of innovation into societal benefits for healthcare services and population health.

Tom Ling

RAND Europe

Tom is Head of Evaluation at RAND Europe and President of the European Evaluation Society, leading evaluations and applied research focused on the key challenges facing health services. His current health portfolio includes evaluations of the innovation landscape, quality improvement, communities of practice, patient flow, and service transformation.

Ellen Perry

THIS Institute (The Healthcare Improvement Studies Institute)

Ellen supported the production of the series during 2020–21.

About the Series

The past decade has seen enormous growth in both activity and research on improvement in healthcare. This series offers a comprehensive and authoritative set of overviews of the different improvement approaches available, exploring the thinking behind them, examining evidence for each approach, and identifying areas of debate.

Cambridge Elements ☰

Improving Quality and Safety in Healthcare

Elements in the Series

A full series listing is available at: www.cambridge.org/IQ

Printed in the United States
by Baker & Taylor Publisher Services